The Body
Restoration Plan

The Body Restoration Plan

ELIMINATE *CHEMICAL CALORIES*™ AND

REPAIR YOUR BODY'S NATURAL

SLIMMING SYSTEM™

Dr. Paula Baillie-Hamilton

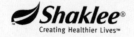

Shaklee®
Creating Healthier Lives™

Copyright © 2002 by Dr. Paula Baillie-Hamilton
Previously published in the U.K. by Michael Joseph as *The Detox Diet*.
Chemical Calorie and *Slimming System* are trademarks of Slimming Systems Ltd.

ISBN 1-58333-166-2

Printed in the United States of America
1   3   5   7   9   10   8   6   4   2

This book is dedicated to the many thousands of scientists world-wide whose vital individual research findings have effectively formed the groundwork from which this book has arisen.

Thank you for reporting the truth as you witnessed it, even if it turned out to be different from the "truth" that you may have been looking for.

Contents

PART FOUR: ACHIEVING A LIFESTYLE THAT MINIMIZES *CHEMICAL CALORIES*

Acknowledgments

No one works in isolation, and this book would never have been possible without the support and help of very many people. I want to start by thanking my entire family, beginning with my husband, Mike. He has helped tremendously, not only by providing continual encouragement and suggestions, but also by providing the financial support that has allowed me free rein to follow and fully develop my ideas. Without his wholehearted support during the last four years, this book would never have seen the light of day.

Likewise, I am indebted to my sister Julia for her helpful review of the manuscript as well as for her extremely constructive advice; to my parents, Pat and John, for teaching me to believe in myself; to my sister Clare for acting as a sounding board; and to my children for making everything worthwhile.

I am also more grateful than I could express to everyone from Shaklee, particularly Dr. Ray Cooper, whom I would particularly like to thank for introducing me to Shaklee and for his unstinting efforts in promoting the book; Cindy Latham for her total enthusiasm every step of the way—Cindy, you are truly inspiring. Special thanks to Terry Kristen Strom for "Americanizing" my book so beautifully. Finally, I would like to thank all those who worked behind the scenes. Their participation was crucial.

Others I would like to thank are:

Fiona Gold, my editor, and her husband, Jonathon, who was one of the first to demonstrate the wonders of the program.

Neeti Madan, my U.S. literary agent from Sterling Lord Literistic, New York, who "got it" immediately and then ran with it.

Laura Shepherd at Penguin Putnam for believing in my book and giving me the benefit of her expert knowledge.

Professor Kim Jobst, who gave me the support and advice I needed to follow my own intuition, and his wife, Belinda, for providing this vital connection.

Dr. Basil Shepstone from Oxford University, my first mentor, who taught me the skills necessary for conducting research as well as gave me great encouragement to continue with my future projects.

Professor Roger Watt and Professor Andrew Watterson, on behalf of and from the Occupational and Environmental Health Research Group at Stirling University, for fully supporting my research.

Elizabeth R. Nesbitt, from the U.S. International Trade Commission, for going beyond the call of duty by kindly photocopying and sending me a huge amount of data from which I created several of my graphs.

Finally, I am extremely grateful to all of the following: Elizabeth McNabb, Sharon Finch, Professor Desmond Hammerton, Professor Vyvyan Howard, Dr. Gera Troisi, Robert Kirby, Neil, Gill, and Alex Baillie-Hamilton, as well as all the other people I have not mentioned who have played a role in supporting me personally or professionally in achieving my goals. Thank you all!

Introduction:
Making the Discovery

I often cast my mind back to how this all began. If I concentrate, I can just about capture a faint impression of myself emerging from the thick fog that had enveloped me following the birth of my second son. I had just snatched a free moment when he was asleep, fallen into a comfy chair, and picked up a newspaper. What drives me so hard to capture that fleeting moment is that, sitting there, I stumbled across the answer to what is arguably one of the greatest unsolved mysteries in medicine today. With hindsight, I recognize that moment to be one of the most significant turning points in my life.

You might very well wonder what on earth was in that newspaper. What caught my eye was an article about the powerful hormone-damaging actions of pesticides, a diverse group of highly toxic chemicals used in food production to kill all kinds of bugs. However, what really grabbed my attention was that the amount of chemicals needed to wreak such havoc with our sex hormones was not too different from the small amount of chemicals we are all exposed to in everyday life.

It just so happened that at the time I was eager to shed some weight and was finding the going pretty tough. After reading the article, it struck me that if these chemicals had the power to alter our hormones so completely, then they must possess some sort of influence on our weight. I made a bee-line for one of my biggest medical textbooks, thumbed through the pages, and there it was in black and white: "Changes in sex hormones can cause weight gain." I was hooked. Three years of uncovering revelation after revelation have resulted in this book. Never in my wildest dreams could I have imagined the sheer wealth of evidence already in the public domain, just waiting to be found.

After I had made the initial connection between toxic chemicals and weight gain, there was no turning back. I can't really explain why I felt so strongly about pursuing the subject, but I felt it then just as strongly as I do now. As every day passed, it became clearer that this was no ordinary finding but a once-in-a-lifetime discovery on the scale that most people only dream about. However, it was also becoming clear that the research necessary to prove such a finding would be fraught with difficulties.

From previous research experience, I knew that a proper investigation would require a serious amount of time and effort as well as easy access to research facilities. The problem was that, for me, life had moved on from the days when I had been working for my scientific doctorate at Christ Church, Oxford. Everything there had been set up for research, the libraries were excellent, and the resources were accessible. Now I was living in a different world. After Oxford, I moved to a rural part of Scotland to become a laird's wife and the proud mother of two young boys. I was completely happy with my new life, but it had become a great deal harder to do any sort of academic work.

If I wanted to consult medical or scientific papers, for example, I couldn't just stroll across the road to one of the world's biggest scientific libraries. I now had to organize a baby-sitter for the boys, make the three-hour round trip to Edinburgh, use the library computer to look up potential papers, spend several hours carting very heavy volumes up and down the stairs to make photocopies of the relevant pages, then rush back home again to read the material. The practical problems slowed everything down, making progress very tough.

As a result, I found myself in a difficult situation. On the one hand, I was desperate to get down to some proper research; on the other, I had major time constraints because of my family and where we lived. Despite the difficulties, however, I was totally gripped by the idea that I had discovered what was causing people to gain weight and by the possibility that my discovery would help millions of people. And as the evidence supporting my ideas stacked up, I was more convinced that giving up was not an option.

Fortunately, this painfully slow research was soon speeded up by a visit from one of my husband's relations, Belinda Jobst. Neither Mike nor I had ever met her before, but it turned out that I had a great deal in common with her husband, Professor Kim Jobst. By a strange coincidence, he is also a medical doctor, had also earned a scientific doctorate from Oxford, and had even been working in Oxford while I was there!

Yet more coincidences followed. He too was very interested in pesticide-free foods and alternative forms of medicine. In fact, he is the editor-in-chief of the *Journal of Alternative and Complementary Medicine*. So I had now come across an expert in the right area, with a background similar to my own in orthodox medicine and science.

The meeting had come at just the right time: I was already feeling the need to talk to someone else about this discovery. Every piece of evidence I had found over the previous months pointed to the conclusion that toxic chemicals were making us fatter. But I recognized that I had been working pretty much in isolation for a long time and that I really needed to hear from someone else that I was on the right track. So one day I told him about my ideas and waited with bated breath to see what he would say. He paused, then smiled and said, "Paula, you have got to write a book about this." This was just the tonic that I needed; there would be no stopping me now!

Hot on the tracks of this encouraging response came the news that it was now possible to access all the scientific information that I needed from the Internet. The National Libraries of America had started to provide free Internet access to Medline, a database of all the medical research papers published worldwide. This was the breakthrough that I needed. Instead of going to Edinburgh, I could now access all the information I needed on my computer at home. My research really took off, as I now had easy access to all the hundreds of thousands of scientific studies that had been published in the past forty years. To everyone at the National Libraries of America—I love you all!

The astonishing fruits of my research, set out in this book, will at last expose the full story behind the tide of excess weight engulfing approximately

Introduction

145 million U.S. citizens and an overall total of 1.2 billion people world-wide.[1] By being led through what has effectively been the last three years of my life, you will discover the primary causes of weight gain and the previously undisclosed key to permanent weight loss in the twenty-first century.

To help guide you through this book, I have divided it into four parts. In Part One, Our Polluted Bodies, I examine the reasons why we are having such a problem with our weight today. Although these initial chapters can be quite detailed at times, they set the scene for the rest of the book. They are full of vital slimming information and advice, making essential reading for all those who want to understand the problem more fully.

In Part Two, I identify the most fattening chemicals in our lives, where they are found in our food and environment, and how to avoid them. The advice I give here should in its own right promote significant weight loss without involving any form of food deprivation—truly effortless weight loss.

Part Three contains vital information about how to safely remove the large quantities of existing fattening chemicals, or *Chemical Calories*, in our bodies, which speeds up the weight loss process and is ideal for those who want to lose weight more quickly.

Finally, in Part Four I tell you how to maintain and enhance your new slimmer figure. I have gotten together with Shaklee in releasing this special Shaklee edition of my book because I truly believe that their products will be of the greatest benefit to you in your quest to lose weight and improve your health. From the very beginning I have been astounded by the similarities between Shaklee's philosophy and mine. As a result, I just love all the products that Shaklee has created! In fact, if I could have designed a company myself from scratch, I could not have come up with a better one than Shaklee. It really seems to have been made for my book!

So if you want to know how you can be part of this major new discovery, which will revolutionize the way we set about losing excess weight, read on. This book will help you, possibly for the first time, achieve your dream of permanent weight loss, improved body shape, and glowing health, virtually effortlessly.

The program has already helped many people lose weight—let it help you too. You will be totally amazed by the results. Say farewell to your excess fat and hello to a new slimmer, fitter, and healthier you.

Part One

OUR POLLUTED BODIES

1

The Fat Epidemic:
Why Are We Still Getting Fatter?

Human beings have unraveled the mysteries of the chromosome, split the atom, walked on the moon, and even taken photographs of the most distant stars in the universe, yet until now we have had no idea what is causing so many of us to become uncomfortably overweight or even dangerously fat. Indeed, many doctors have publicly admitted defeat, effectively raising the white flag in the battle of the bulge.[1]

The situation has become so bad that leading doctors have suggested that much of the Western world is gripped by a full-blown fatness epidemic. William Dietz, the director of nutrition at the Center for Disease Control, certainly pulled no punches when he said in 1999: "This is an epidemic in the U.S., the likes of which we have not had before in chronic disease."[2] Another leading scientist, James Hill, Dean of American obesity studies at the University of Colorado, has gone so far as to say that if the fat epidemic is not checked, most Americans will be overweight within a few generations.[3]

What makes the situation even worse is that our children appear to be increasingly at risk for obesity.[4] This has set loud alarm bells ringing, since it is well known that overweight children are far more likely to stay overweight throughout their adult lives.

7

We already know that the depressing trend for adults is to get heavier as they get older. Current estimates suggest that the average woman gains approximately one pound each year and the average man gains one-half pound.[5]

It's not too difficult to believe these frightening figures—just take a look around, and you can see for yourself. More people are overweight now than ever before. Even seats in public places are being replaced because they are no longer wide enough for many Americans.

Our Body Shape Is Changing Too

But it doesn't stop at our weight: It is increasingly apparent that even our basic body shape seems to be changing. Women are gaining more weight around the abdomen and hips and are also developing bigger busts.[6] Men are becoming more rotund, particularly around the waist. These relentless increases in weight and ballooning shapes have been so dramatic that the standard clothing sizes used for the last fifty years have had to be scrapped and completely revamped.[7]

An experienced underwear fitter I met recently confirmed this. She told me that when she started her career forty years ago, a DD bra fitting was extremely uncommon and an E fitting simply didn't exist. Now DD and E fittings are among the most common bra sizes she sells!

Dieting Alone Simply Doesn't Work!

Somewhat incomprehensibly, our battle with our weight seems to grow and grow in spite of our best efforts to stem the tide. Yet the harder we try, the less effective our efforts seem to be. Surely, if traditional dieting methods really worked, the fat epidemic should have been stamped out long ago. Granted, in the short term, many people do lose weight by sticking to a particular diet or regime. But the overwhelming evidence is that they will regain all the weight lost, and then some more, as soon as they return to "normal life."[8]

However, that's by no means the end of the bad news. For when you diet, the proportion of lean muscular tissue you possess dramatically falls while the proportion of your body fat greatly increases, producing a disastrous effect on your overall body shape.[9] Then when you regain the weight you have lost, the body gains fat in preference to lean muscle, so you end up with a greater proportion of body fat than when you first started.

For many people, the final reward for all those weeks or months of deprivation and exertion is that they are likely to end up being fatter and more out of shape than they would have been if they had put on more weight just by overeating! To add insult to injury, by the time you are driven to try the next new diet, your excess weight will be that much harder to shift.

So not only do most diets not work, but there is increasing evidence that they are actually making us fatter!

Being Overweight Destroys Self-esteem

The harsh reality is that as long as there is widespread prejudice against those who are overweight, most people will ignore all the evidence and keep on trying diet after diet to try to reach their ideal body weight. The motivation to be slim is extremely powerful and should never be underestimated.

Magazines, film, and television all promote images of people who are unrealistically skinny. But because of their powerful influence on our society, the message accepted by most people is that this is the shape people have to be if they want to be considered attractive or lovable.

The flip side of this message is considerably more negative, with fatter people being labeled as either greedy or lazy. Since overindulgence and laziness are signs of weakness in our society, being seriously overweight is considered a massive social stigma, a self-inflicted and ugly problem eliciting very little sympathy or understanding.

Like it or not, appearance plays a very important part in how we relate to others and how they react to us. Society treats overweight people very differently from their slimmer counterparts. Overweight children often bear the brunt of teasing in the classroom and can become withdrawn, developing fewer social skills. With adults the effects are subtler, such as not being selected for a job or having more difficulty finding a partner. This can cause people to remove themselves from many situations, particularly high-profile or intimate situations in which they would be visible or exposed.

For many of us, it's only a matter of losing a few pounds to reach our ideal weight; for others, being overweight can take a huge personal toll on our lives, driving us to seek ever more desperate ways of losing that unwanted fat. Indeed, many people would do virtually anything to achieve their goal, such as putting themselves through major operations and treatments, with the accompanying pain and risks, in an attempt to become slimmer.

Public Health Enemy No. 1

But it's not just our appearance that is at stake. Life-threatening illnesses such as heart disease, diabetes, cancer, and strokes are all closely linked to being overweight, and their incidences are all on the increase. Excessive weight is swiftly developing into public health enemy No. 1, not just because of the problems it causes in its own right but because of all the other illnesses that accompany it.[10]

Yet being overweight is not the only factor behind the higher rates of illness suffered by overweight people. Research has shown that people whose weight "yo-yos" from one extreme to the other can have up to double the death rate from all forms of illness (particularly diabetes and heart disease) compared to that of those whose weight remains stable.[11] So if people try to tackle their weight and health problems by traditional dieting methods, they can unwittingly put their own health at risk.

Before I leave this serious subject, there is one more aspect to the fat epidemic, one that sends shivers down the spines of hospital administrators and politicians: It is the cost to the nation of treating overweight- and fat-related problems. In the United Kingdom this cost is currently estimated at more than $3 billion every year and in the United States at a massive $68 billion.[12] And, as the years go on, these figures keep growing. So to have any chance of dealing with the rising tide of illness, governments are now being forced to become more and more involved with these issues, treating the fat epidemic as a national health problem as well as a personal challenge for millions of people.

Unfortunately, the authorities currently are helpless; until they fully understand the cause of excessive weight gain, they can offer us no new answers. Their best recommendation is that we should eat less and exercise more. Well, what do they think the majority of us have been trying to do all these years?

The Fat Epidemic Is a Very Recent Phenomenon

Why are we still getting fatter? With untold sums being spent every year on trying to lose weight, the last thing we want to hear is that there is no cure. Despite increased awareness, buying of low-calorie foods, and booming membership of fitness clubs, we are becoming fatter than ever. What on earth is going on?

To understand the situation, we need to look back to the time before our weight began to be such a huge problem. Take a look at Figure 1, which tracks weight gain throughout the last half-century. You can see that the increase in the number of overweight people was initially very slow and consistent in the '60s and '70s, but that suddenly in the '80s and '90s the numbers rocketed.[13] This graph reveals that we are not just dealing with a gradual trickle of cases but are in the grip of a totally new phenomenon.

To understand still more about our current predicament, we now need to look back to our dieting past to get more of a feel for what factors could be behind the present problem.

A Brief History of Dieting

The next time you see an old black-and-white film or flip through old photos in your family album, count how many people are overweight. There will be a few, certainly, but the problem was on a much smaller scale than it is

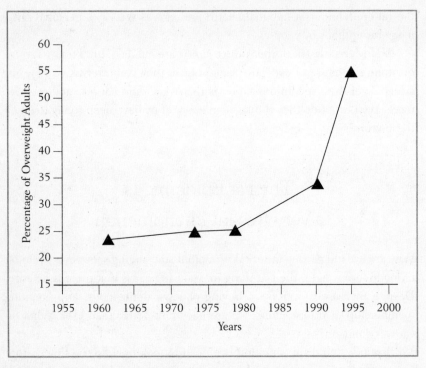

Figure 1. The percentage of overweight U.S. adults over recent years

today. In truth, dieting as we recognize it today didn't even exist until about midway through the twentieth century. Before then, excess weight had been treated by fasting or by other methods, such as nibbling on soap or taking laxatives.

All this changed with the conception of the food restriction "diet" by Drs. Johnston and Newburgh in the 1930s at the University of Michigan. Their theory was simple and is well known by most people today. If a person consumes fewer calories than his or her body burns, then the body will burn its fat stores to make up the energy deficit. This simplistic theory has provided the basis for most of the thousands of diet books written since then, which basically differ from each other only by fiddling about with the proportions of fats, carbohydrates, and proteins that they allow.

As the number of overweight people continued to increase through the '40s and '50s, more people started asking for expert help. It seemed as if the natural checks and balances that had served us for centuries didn't work anymore.

One of the first diet "bibles" was *The Slimming Business,* written by the nutritionist Professor John Yudkin and published in 1958. He recommended a diet very low in carbohydrates, with higher levels of fat-rich foods, which is actually very similar to the low-carbohydrate diets popular today. Very-low-carbohydrate diets were found to induce an abnormal metabolic state known as *ketosis*[14] as well as mood changes, carbohydrate cravings, and irritability. Even if dieters were prepared to risk these side effects, low-carbohydrate eating also caused the body to accumulate fat more quickly when people came off the diet.

In the '70s, very-low-calorie diets, or "crash diets," came into fashion, encouraging dieters to stick to about 1,000 calories a day. This form of dieting soon fell from favor because it made people lose both muscle and fat, and it did not change their long-term eating habits. So any weight lost was regained very quickly.

Possibly the best-selling diet book ever written was *The Complete Scarsdale Medical Diet,* by Dr. Herman Tarnower, published in 1978.[15] It was the first diet I ever went on, and my lasting memories of it are painful to say the least. Fundamentally it was a high-protein/low-carbohydrate diet, and it did help me lose weight temporarily. However, the gastric side effects from eating vast quantities of onions, carrots, cabbage, and tomatoes, which were often the only foods allowed to be eaten freely, were unreal.

It was followed in the '80s by Judy Mazel's glitzy *The Beverly Hills Diet,* which was based on the food-combining theory of eating proteins and carbohydrates separately. Because of its nickname, "the diarrhea diet," I decided not to use this diet to remove the pounds I had regained following the Scarsdale Diet. I was most definitely not going to do anything that upsets my gut again!

The '90s were hit by Barry Sears's very fashionable *Enter the Zone,* which recommends a low-carbohydrate and high-protein intake.[16] Recently, more books promoting low-carbohydrate eating have been released, most notably Dr. Atkins's *New Diet Revolution.*[17] These are a variation on the earlier diet books of the '50s, so fashion appears to have come round full circle.

Yet despite the attractiveness of the concept, it now seems pretty clear that no amount of fiddling with proportions of food alone can result in a permanent solution. There is, however, one possible answer that could explain why our weight problems are becoming more prominent, but its implications are very serious indeed. It could be that our bodies are losing their natural ability to regulate their own weight.

Solving the Greatest Twenty-First-Century Mystery

The ability to control body weight is one of the most fundamental and highly developed of all our bodily functions. It has evolved over many hundreds of thousands of years, allowing our bodies to adapt and survive through different environmental stresses, such as famine and drought, as well as times of plenty.[18]

For many of our ancestors, size was literally a matter of life or death. If you were too fat, it reduced your ability to hunt effectively or flee from the occasional saber-toothed wildcat that came your way. If too thin, you could perish. Survival of the fittest ensured that those who could adapt to different situations would be the winners. If something is indeed poisoning our weight control mechanisms then, until it is identified, no amount of dieting will ever make us lose weight. So what could be causing it?

Well, we need to go back to the basics of whether a problem is inherited or acquired. The time needed for a change in our genetic makeup big enough to have brought about this fat epidemic is thousands of years. Since, as we can clearly see from Figure 1, the problem has largely occurred during a couple of decades, this cause can effectively be ruled out. So the potential cause can be narrowed down to changes in our environment or our lifestyles.

Could there be a way in which our environment or the way we live has significantly changed in the past century? And could this change have caused a fundamental difference in the way our weight control systems work?

Unfortunately, the answer is yes. During this century, we have been exposed to substances that have been shown to cause profound damage to all the systems involved in weight control. So powerful does this "fattening" effect appear to be that it has resulted in many of these substances actually being widely used in agriculture to fatten up animals. They have been used in medicine to help underweight individuals gain weight.

These substances are used on a vast scale and cause damage at the levels at which they are currently found in the environment.[19] Their use has been so insidious that we have hardly noticed. Their manufacture has grown from nothing to a multibillion-dollar-a-year industry worldwide.[20] Considered essential by most who use them, these substances have changed the practice of farming and industry to such an extent that life without them now is almost unthinkable. Yet they have only been around for a very short time.

What are they?

Man-made chemicals.

2

The Synthetic Revolution:
How Toxic Chemicals
Have Invaded Our Bodies

In this chapter you will discover how the production of man-made, or synthetic, chemicals has in some way touched everybody's lives. Since their first creation more than 150 years ago, these substances have been produced in increasingly massive quantities and appear to have the ability to contaminate and damage both wildlife and humans. Yet most people, and even the majority of doctors, seem to know next to nothing about what is going on in their environment and indeed, more specifically, underneath their very own skin.

In trying to explain the sheer enormity of the problem we all now face from this chemical onslaught, we need to know a bit more about the current size of the problem, the ways in which these chemicals compromise our health, what sorts of substances are involved, and just why they cause such extreme havoc to our body weight and well-being.

I can fully appreciate that much of the information in this chapter may be worrying. But you have to realize that by understanding the issues, you will be one short step away from dealing with them. Don't become too alarmed, since the rest of the book will contain the ground rules for simple ways to help your body deal effectively with the new polluted environment in which we now find ourselves living.

By following the advice contained in this book, you will get all the relevant know-how you need to lose weight and thrive in the twenty-first century! But if time is short and you want to know now which chemicals are making us fatter and where they are found, you could skip this chapter and go straight to Chapter 3, then come back to this one when you have more time.

From No Exposure to Overexposure

The creation and widespread use of toxic synthetic chemicals in the late twentieth century has permanently changed the face of our planet. As a result, every single region of the planet has been permanently contaminated with a cocktail of toxins. Whether you go to the North Pole or to the desert, these toxins can now be found everywhere.[1]

Don't make the mistake of thinking that the only people at risk are those who are exposed to them at work, for in this man-made polluted environment in which we all now live, every last one of us is bombarded on a daily basis by massive amounts of these chemicals. OK, admittedly few people deliberately set out to expose themselves to these toxins, but the simple act of eating certain contaminated foods or using certain "treated" products could be putting you at risk without your even realizing it.

And don't think that just because you can't see them, they are not there. After all, the many hundreds of billions of pounds of these synthetic chemicals produced every single year have to go somewhere!

We end up eating these chemicals in our foods as pesticides, preservatives, additives, pollutants, and contaminants from food containers. We drink them in tap water, which contains chemicals leached from contaminated soils, environmental pollutants, and even chemicals added deliberately. We absorb them though our skin from cosmetics, toiletries, treated wood, sprayed plants, and treated areas of public parks, golf courses, and swimming pools. We even inhale them in air contaminated with solvents, car fumes, industrial waste, and environmental pollutants. As you can see, there are very few places left to hide.

The Extent to Which We Are
Now Contaminated

It has been calculated that one new chemical enters industrial use every twenty minutes, and many hundreds of thousands of them are already out there.[2] As a result, the average person living in the developed world is now contaminated with up to 500 industrial toxins, few of which have been properly tested for harmful effects.[3]

Dr. Steven Stellman at the American Health Foundation in New York found significant levels of organochlorines (one of the most poisonous and persistent kinds of toxic chemicals known to man) in the fat tissue of women who lived in Long Island, New York.[4] Shockingly, the levels at which they were detected were not just double or triple the levels commonly found in animal fat products, but were approximately twenty-four times higher than the levels found in the most polluted type of animal fat tested, in this case butter.[5]

The stark truth is that apparently, despite many of us not realizing it, we are all so polluted that if we were cannibals, our meat would most certainly be unfit for human consumption!

The Growing Link Between
Chemicals and Disease

As every year passes, it becomes more and more apparent that the introduction of these highly toxic chemicals into our lives has resulted in setting off a disease time bomb. It now seems that a staggeringly large number of the most common diseases of the developed world are related to or can be triggered by these toxins. This list includes most kinds of cancer, hormonal disorders, low energy levels, chronic fatigue syndrome, sexual problems, immune disorders, and heart disease.[6]

So What Are These Chemicals?

The chemicals that appear to be causing all these problems can basically be divided into two main groups: toxic heavy metals and synthetic chemicals.

Toxic heavy metals, which include substances such as lead, cadmium, mercury, and manganese, have been around as long as we have, since they are part of our natural world. The problem is that, due to the explosive increase in manufacturing, we are now exposed to levels far higher than our bodies were ever designed to withstand. As a result, these unnaturally high levels have been found to cause a whole range of health problems, such as impaired intelligence and permanent nerve damage, as well as to trigger a number of other diseases.[7]

Synthetic chemicals are definitely not natural, since they are all manufactured in chemical laboratories. Because of the massive quantities produced, along with their widespread use and potential for excessive toxicity, they appear to be the main troublemakers. In addition, unlike the heavy metals, which we have developed some mechanisms for dealing with over the years, we simply have no way of dealing with many of these chemicals, and many of them just end up accumulating in our bodies.

Synthetic Chemicals

Synthetic chemicals are an extremely big business. Production in the United States alone in 1994 was worth a staggering $101 billion, and Figure 2 shows the phenomenal increase in production of these substances throughout the twentieth century.[8]

We use synthetic chemicals in pesticides, solvents, dyes, medicines, industrial chemicals, rubber, food preservatives, and many other products. Because more uses for new chemicals are being found, the quantities produced keep increasing. This has seriously affected the markets for more traditional materials, which as a direct result are becoming less and less popular. Think about it: When was the last time you bought milk in a glass bottle?

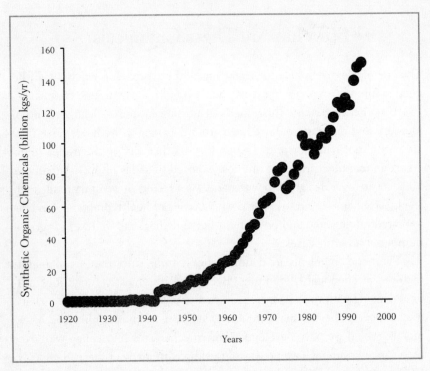

Figure 2. The annual U.S. production of synthetic chemicals in the twentieth century

Why Do We Use Synthetic Chemicals?

To get to the bottom of why synthetic chemicals are so widely preferred to naturally occurring substances, we need to know a bit more about them and what makes them so popular with manufacturers.

It may surprise some, but most synthetic chemicals are actually derived from natural substances, usually either crude oil or coal, which themselves are the products of organisms that lived many thousands of years ago. During the industrial revolution in the nineteenth century, we discovered how to convert crude oil and coal into synthetic chemicals by subjecting them to extreme temperatures, among other methods. What happens is that the molecules of the natural oil or coal tar are manipulated and rearranged into an entirely new structure that simply does not occur in nature.

With this new structure often comes a whole new set of properties, such as increased stability, increased longevity, high toxicity, and reduced biodegradability. These new qualities are the reasons synthetic substances are so widely used, as in many cases they can offer clear advantages over natural materials.[9] For instance, why buy wooden window frames that need to be painted regularly when you could buy lower-maintenance synthetic ones instead?

As a result, since we first discovered these man-made substances, research has been intense to identify new compounds that possess even more "beneficial" qualities. And so hundreds of thousands of synthetic chemicals have now been created, each with its own particular properties.

Chemicals that are extremely stable can be used as fire retardants or insulators. Chemicals that powerfully manipulate our bodily functions tend to be used as medicines, for both humans and animals, or as pesticides to kill insects as well as many other forms of life. Chemicals that possess strong colors are used as pigments or food colorings; chemicals that add malleability are used to make synthetic materials flexible.

Unnatural Properties Create New Problems

Because the raw ingredients of synthetic chemicals (oil and coal) are the products of fossilized plants and animals, these new synthetic substances are made up of the same molecules that were found in once-living creatures. This makes the new chemicals similar enough to natural materials to be recognized by our bodies. However, their new properties (increased stability, different structures, and so on) make them act in a completely unnatural way, which is in fact the very heart of the problem.

On the one hand, this similarity to naturally produced substances allows them to be assimilated into many of our body's natural processes, including all the systems essential in supporting animal life.[10] In other words, synthetic chemicals can mimic natural substances and can fool the body into carrying out certain functions, and so be very useful, for example, as medicines.

On the other hand, because of their different shapes and increased stability, they do not react in the same way as natural substances, which tend to break down or are switched off after having completed their work. As a result, many synthetic compounds do not break down or get "switched off" after performing their function.[11] Instead, they can keep on falsely stimulating or disrupting our bodies twenty-four hours a day, seven days a week. This low-grade but continual long-term damage to many of our body's systems is precisely why they appear to pose such a major problem to our health.

Our Bodies Are Not Designed to Cope with Synthetic Chemicals

Over millions of years, our bodies have developed very sophisticated detoxification systems to rid themselves of most naturally produced toxins on a day-to-day basis. (There are plenty of different natural toxins in our environment, such as certain fungi and bacteria.) The problem is that these new artificial compounds have structures totally alien to our highly developed detoxification systems, as our bodies have not been confronted with them in the past. As a result, our waste-disposal systems can manage to process some of these "alien" chemicals but often fail miserably in dealing with others. This results in a buildup of certain toxic chemicals in our body.[12]

In effect, most of the chemicals that we cannot eliminate end up being stored in our adipose tissue (body fat) due to their high fat solubility. Contrary to popular belief, however, once in the fat stores they are not out of harm's way, because once there they set to work damaging our fat metabolism.[13]

If there were some way in which we could break down many of these chemicals into more harmless products, they would not be so dangerous. But because some are so untouchable, our bodies cannot get rid of them, and so they keep on accumulating throughout our lives.[14]

We Need to Adapt to Survive

It is also becoming clearer that people whose systems are better able to deal with these chemicals are far less prone to chemical-related problems than are others.[15] Darwinian theories hold true here. Those who are better able to adjust to their new environmental conditions will pull through in the survival of the fittest. So what makes some people better able to process these chemicals than others?

Well, the first important factor is the current state of nutrition. The additional work caused by our bodies' efforts to process these new chemicals has resulted in a "devitaminizing effect." In other words, our bodies are now using up certain vitamin supplies more rapidly than we have probably ever done in our history. So the presence of these chemicals has had the effect of considerably increasing our requirement not only for these vitamins but also for all the other nutrients that are vital in processing these toxic substances.[16] Thus for all intents and purposes, the presence of artificial chemicals has permanently increased our overall nutritional needs. Those people who have a better level of nutrition will possess a greater ability to process these chemicals than will those whose diets and nutritional supplements are inferior.

But it is not just the state of nutrition that determines an individual's ability to deal with these chemicals; a whole range of other factors, such as genetic predisposition, age,[17] level of exposure, and even dieting history,[18] have their own influences.

The bottom line is that the more able people are to rid their bodies of these chemicals, the less susceptible they will be to piling on the pounds and the less likely to develop a whole range of chemical-related illnesses. The key is to discover how to adapt to our new environment. That is the essence of this book.

How Do These Chemicals Enter Our Bodies?

So how do these chemicals actually enter our bodies? The main way is through our food and drink, but they are also readily absorbed through the skin and breathed in through the lungs.

Rather than discussing this now, I will limit the discussion in the rest of this chapter to explaining the main ways in which our intake of chemicals has increased via our food.

The Origins of "Conventional" Farming in the Twentieth Century

After the creation of synthetic chemicals at the end of the nineteenth century, scientists found that certain compounds possessed a deadly ability to interfere with many of the vital processes essential for life, so much so that even the tiniest amounts of these substances could kill virtually any life form. This was a gift to the authorities who realized their potential for chemical warfare and developed it. But after the Second World War was over, they needed to find other uses for these substances, which they were now producing in ever-increasing quantities. It was then that these deadly chemicals started to be used as pesticides in the farming community.

It soon became clear that these new pesticides at lower concentrations were just as good at killing insects as were higher levels designed to kill humans. So it made good economic sense to farmers to use them in reducing the pest damage to their crops. In fact, these "wonder" chemicals were so effective that, before long, chemical pest control had spread throughout the international farming community with breathtaking speed, changing the way we farmed beyond all recognition. This new way is now known as *conventional farming*.

Chemicals Are Poisoning Our Foods

As a result of this fundamental change to the way we now farm, most of the food we eat today has been sprayed with all kinds of highly toxic chemicals designed to kill insects (insecticides), fungus (fungicides), bacteria (antibacterials), animals (rodenticides), and weeds (herbicides). Collectively these are all known as pesticides. After your food is harvested, it may be sprayed again to prevent it from going bad in storage. And before it is packaged, it may be treated with yet more chemicals.

Apples and strawberries are commonly sprayed with a large number of pesticides while they are growing. For example, in one batch of food tested by the FDA, eight different kinds of pesticide residues were found on a sample of apples, and nine different pesticides were identified on strawberries.[19] Even processed foods can have chemicals deliberately added to them to increase their shelf life. As a result of these and other practices, approximately two-thirds of the foods we eat have some detectable amount of deliberately added pesticides or chemicals still on them.[20]

This is a totally unnatural state of affairs. Never before has food contained these destructive toxins, all of which have been designed to kill. By carrying on in this way, we are effectively poisoning our food supplies and with them ourselves.

But because of the widespread contamination of our environment, our food is contaminated not only by the pesticides that are deliberately added to it but also by a whole raft of industrial waste products present in food packaging, the air, water, and soil. So by the time your food gets to you, not only will it contain the ingredients listed on the label, but chances are it will contain an awful lot more.

Now that I have set the scene by introducing you to the many problems that exposure to these chemicals has created, it is time to give you what you really want to know. So sit back, turn the page, and you will discover for yourself the startling evidence supporting my discovery that these toxic chemicals appear to be making us all fatter.

3

Chemicals That Make You Fat: The Medical Evidence

When I started researching this book, never in a million years did I expect to find the overwhelming evidence that I've now uncovered. The solution to the puzzle of why we are all becoming fatter is under our very noses. It lurks in every bite of food we eat, in every sip of liquid we drink, and in the very air we breathe. Now the time has come for the evidence to be pieced together. I think the easiest way to explain the growing problem of obesity is to use a simple financial example.

Chemicals Cause Weight Gain

Imagine a beef farmer who raises cattle and sells them for slaughter. One of his major expenses will be animal feed, and his profit will depend on the final weight of the cattle. The more it costs him to feed the cattle, the less profit he will make. If he had a magic "fattening" pill, his cows would eat less food and put on more weight, so he would make more money. It is therefore not surprising that farmers have actually been using powerful synthetic fattening chemicals for a long time to enhance animal weight gain.

For example, since 1976, the increasing use of growth-promoting feed additives, selective breeding, and high-protein diets has reduced the amount of feed needed for broiler chickens to reach a better market size by almost 40 percent.[1]

The way that most of these chemicals act is to greatly improve food efficiency; in other words, they alter the animals' metabolism so that less food goes much further. Animals that eat these chemicals in their feed end up gaining more weight than untreated animals, even when the untreated animals are eating *more* food.[2] It makes total economic sense. More animal weight for less food. Feed bills are reduced, and income is increased because the farmer will get a better price at market. And after the animals are sold, guess what? We eat them, chemicals and all.

Synthetic Chemicals Are Making Us Fat

Our metabolism appears to be affected by a massive range of synthetic chemicals—in all probability including those intended to "fatten" animals—in a very similar way. Different synthetic chemicals achieve this effect in humans and other mammals in one or more ways. First they appear to damage the appetite "switch," so that we eat more food than we generally need.[3] In addition, they reduce the amount of food our body needs by damaging its ability to burn off food, thereby making the food we eat go further.[4] But possibly the most important way these chemicals function is by seemingly preventing the body from burning up existing fat stores.[5]

So, in effect, many synthetic chemicals appear to possess the potential to poison critical parts of our weight control system, effectively putting it out of action. What's worse, unless properly tackled, the effect could be cumulative or even synergistic, dooming us to become fatter and fatter as long as we keep exposing our bodies to these chemicals.

At this point I think it would be very useful to look at how the time scale of the fat epidemic relates to the increased production of synthetic chemicals. Figure 3 shows the relationship between the rising production of synthetic chemicals in America and the rise in the percentage of U.S. adults who are overweight.[6,7]

You can see for yourself that the explosion in the production of syn-

The Body Restoration Plan

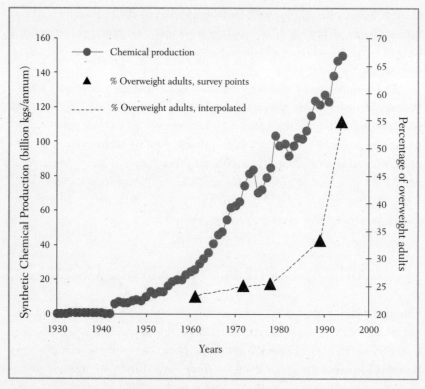

Figure 3. The increase in number of overweight U.S. adults and the increase in the U.S. production of synthetic chemicals over the twentieth century

thetic chemicals precedes an equally dramatic recent rise in the number of people who are becoming overweight. The very speed of the recent marked increases in the number of overweight people indicates that changes in the environment are far more likely to be the source of the problem than genetic changes, which would take much longer to occur. This time scale would also fit with chemicals being the cause of the fat epidemic.

Although the graph in itself does not prove that the two are linked, it certainly gives an indication that this suggestion is plausible. The fact that synthetic chemicals are actually known to cause weight gain provides additional support for my ideas.

So, considering the ever-increasing amounts of these chemicals that we are being exposed to in our lives, is it surprising that it has been said that excessive weight gain is becoming a normal response to the American environment?

This would also explain why simple food-restriction dieting simply does not work for many of us over the long term, as it totally fails to deal with removing fattening chemicals from our lives. Their removal is a vital part of tackling the problem.

So Where Is the Proof That These Chemicals Can Make Us Fat?

In making the revolutionary claim that our exposure to synthetic chemicals is at the heart of the current fat epidemic, it is vital to be able to back the statement up with evidence. So when I started my investigations, I spent many months scouring medical and scientific libraries, gathering together hundreds of academic papers that could help me get a grip on what was happening.

My medical specialty and scientific background kicked in here, enabling me to ask the right questions and begin getting pieces of the answer. But it was only toward the end of this lengthy and thorough process that the full picture gradually but spectacularly fell into place.

These papers revealed how growth promoters, pesticides,[8] synthetics,[9] toxic chemicals,[10] and a whole range of the most common environmental pollutants around us[11] produce fattening effects in animals and humans. In plain English, I discovered that these chemicals appear to be making us fat.

The sheer number of fattening chemicals in our environment meant that it took me more than a year to get all my evidence together. Every step of the way, I kept making new discoveries that confirmed my initial suspicions. Time and time again, when I learned about a different group of pesticides or environmental pollutants, I would soon discover that they too could cause weight gain.

If It's Poisonous, It Should Cause Weight Loss, Not Gain!

So, you may well ask, if all the evidence is already there, why has it taken so long to come to light? Until very recently, scientists have believed that because pesticides and other synthetic chemicals are toxic, their only possible effect on weight could be one of weight loss.[12] I suppose this prejudice was not so surprising: Large doses of chemicals are indeed extremely toxic and tend to cause those affected to become very ill, and when you are feeling dreadful, you don't have much of an appetite. The weight-gain effect that I uncovered is found at the other end of the exposure spectrum, where the person or animal is exposed to extremely low doses of chemicals. At these low levels, the weight control systems are still damaged, but the person or animal doesn't actually feel ill and stop eating.

The main problem I had in finding my evidence resulted directly from the general assumption that these synthetic chemicals would cause weight loss. Studies designed to assess the toxicity of a chemical that found weight gain rather than weight loss tended to ignore the finding as irrelevant to the study or try to dismiss the finding. I even found one report, investigating the toxicity of synthetic materials, that actually apologized for finding weight gain, as it was not at all what the scientists had hoped for![13] In addition, weight gains were not reported in the summaries of many earlier scientific papers, making it impossible to determine whether a study showed a weight gain effect or not by searching modern scientific databases, which contain only information extracted from the summaries. Although more recently scientists have accepted that chemicals *can* cause weight gain,[14] the fuller picture simply has not been seen until now because of the difficulty of retrieving much of this "hidden" evidence from the past.

I was so convinced that a weight-gain effect was happening that I spent a huge amount of time ordering up complete copies of these scientific papers, in the hope that a few of them would reveal these weight-gain effects. Typically, one study out of every ten of the papers I had ordered had used doses low enough to reveal this weight-gain effect. Every time I found one of these precious papers showing that yet another major group of chemicals produced weight gain, I was absolutely elated!

These numerous small but highly significant discoveries over time were essential in strengthening my ideas and spurred me on to uncover the whole picture. The more I delved into the subject, the more extensive and conclusive the evidence became. Reflecting on the situation, if I had simply accepted the easily accessible summaries at face value and not actually spent months retrieving and reading the full original papers, this book never would have been written.

The Chemicals That Make People Fat Are All Around Us

With hundreds of thousands of synthetic chemicals already out there, and with a new substance being introduced into industrial usage every twenty minutes, I needed some way to simplify my research. So, rather than looking at each chemical individually, which would have been virtually impossible, I grouped the chemicals together according to their structure. This approach soon proved invaluable, as it opened my eyes to the discovery that one type of chemical can actually have many different uses.

This became more and more apparent as I went through each one of the dozens of different synthetic chemicals found as pesticide residues in food. It rapidly became clear that the same chemicals or some that are very similar to ones that were being used to kill a huge variety of different life forms and to promote growth in animals[15] were associated with weight gain in humans[16] and were even regularly used as medicines to treat a whole range of human illnesses.[17]

But it didn't stop there: I also discovered that the same or similar chemicals were also widely used in a huge range of cosmetics, toiletries, and other household products. In other words, we are being exposed to these fattening chemicals in a whole variety of ways.

So what are these chemicals? Well, there is a broad range of chemicals that cause weight gain, including pesticides, medicines, heavy metals,[18] synthetic materials,[19] solvents, environmental pollutants, fire retardants,[20] and many other substances. Because of the sheer number of chemicals I have found with fattening effects, it would be far too confusing to deal with all of them at once. So I have decided to highlight just those chemicals that are actually used to promote fattening in animals.

Following this, I will expose some of the human evidence showing that chemically induced weight gain can be deliberately induced on occasions but is more commonly an unwanted side effect of many synthetic medications. After that, I will explain how certain persistent chemicals are already present in some of us at levels that appear to be making us fatter.

The Animal Growth Promoters

When I found the first paper showing that one of the most commonly detected pesticides in our food was also actually used as a growth promoter to fatten up animals, I knew I was on to something. It's one thing to find that chemicals have a fattening effect on animals but quite another to discover that they have been deliberately used for this purpose in real life. Suddenly the whole thing changed from a hypothesis into reality. The extensive group of substances that I am about to describe proves, I believe, beyond reasonable doubt that chemicals can make you fat, because they have been used for precisely this purpose for many years.

Although some of these growth promoters are now banned from this particular use, we are still being exposed to most of them, both as pesticides in our food and in many other products commonly used around the home and in our environment. So which are the worst offenders, and where else can these substances be found?

ORGANOPHOSPHATES

The organophosphates are particularly good examples of "fattening" synthetic chemicals. They were initially developed for use in human warfare. Later it was discovered that as well as being highly toxic to humans, they are also very effective at killing insects. This discovery led to their extensive use on food crops, and now they are some of the most common pesticides found in our soft fruit and vegetables.

However, what really struck me about organophosphates was that this same group of chemicals had another commercial use: to fatten up livestock! Although many studies had shown that organophosphates possessed a marked fattening effect, to discover that they were actually used for this purpose really drove my point home. What made it even worse was that the same type of chemical used to fatten up cattle (at very low doses) was also found on our food (again in very low doses) because of its use as a crop insecticide. It could even be found in many other products, for example, flea powders and household fly spray.[21]

So how does this group of chemicals promote fattening? Well, at low doses, organophosphates appear to fatten up cows by severely reducing their ability to use up existing fat stores. As the animals' fat-burning abilities slow down, they gain weight more quickly, since they just can't burn off body fat as well as they previously could. Their food needs also fall, as less food appears to go further. Though the use of organophosphates as growth promoters has now been banned, they are still one of the most common pesticides used in the production of many of our foods. They are also commonly used in the manufacture of rubber and other synthetic materials, in gasoline as additives, and in lubricating oils.

It really doesn't matter how you are exposed, whether it is from a can of fly spray or from pesticide residues in food. Once organophosphates get into your body, chances are they will proceed to damage your weight control systems, making it just that little bit harder to lose weight in the future.

While I am on the subject of organophosphates, I must mention their toxic effects on the nerves and muscles (remember, they were originally developed to be used as nerve gas). When I was working as a hospital doctor, there was an incident that really shocked me at the time, and to this day I can remember it quite clearly. We got a call about a person who had deliberately swallowed a teaspoon of household pesticide. We had no idea what chemicals were in the poison and just had to wait until the ambulance appeared.

Virtually the first thing the patient did after being wheeled into the casualty department was to stop breathing. This was followed by continual violent convulsions, and it took a whole team of us several hours to stabilize the patient in intensive care. When coming to a few days later, the patient's muscles were extremely weak, to such an extent that he could barely lift his head from the pillow. It turned out that organophosphate was the main active ingredient in the pesticide.

It is this extreme damage to the muscles that I want to highlight here. As well as having the ability to reduce and slow down fat metabolism, organophosphates can seriously impair a person's ability to exercise. They can permanently damage nerves,[22] break down the structure of muscle fibers, reduce the ability to produce energy to power exercise, and, to cap it all, reduce the desire to exercise.[23] This powerful ability to lower exercise levels makes organophosphates even better growth promoters, as exposed animals that exercise less will use up fewer calories. Remember that the next time you think about wielding a can of fly spray.

CARBAMATES

Carbamates are some of the most widely used chemicals in agriculture. In addition to being used as common insecticides for crops such as tobacco and cotton and as a treatment for wood infestations, they are also used in large quantities in an extensive range of foods, including potatoes, peanuts, and citrus fruit, along with many other fruits and vegetables, as fungicides (when they are more commonly known as bisthiocarbamates). Because fungicides tend to be added to foods close to harvest, there is less opportunity for them to be washed off by the rain. As a result, carbamates can often be found in relatively high levels in food.

As well as being commonly used as pesticides, certain kinds of carbamates possess extremely powerful fattening abilities, which, in combination with their antibacterial properties, have resulted in their widespread use in animal husbandry. The main way in which they are thought to cause fattening is by reducing the overall metabolic rate, in essence making less food go further.[24] In addition they, like the organophosphates, can also lower the overall level of physical activity.[25] The irony is that most people eating fruit and vegetables treated with these chemicals would think they had chosen low-fat healthy foods to help them keep their weight down!

THYROID DRUGS

Some of the most critical hormones our bodies use to burn off excess weight are the thyroid hormones. So it is not surprising that several chemicals designed to suppress the production of this potent fat-burning hormone have been used as growth promoters because of their ability to make animals pile on the fat.[26] Although all these thyroid-hormone-suppressing or "antithyroid" compounds are now banned for this use, similar compounds are still being commonly found on our foods as pesticides.

We definitely know that they also cause weight gain in humans, as these antithyroid substances are commonly used in humans to suppress overactive thyroid disease.[27] If too large a dose is given, it causes excess weight gain.

However, it gets worse: I have found that not only do a couple of chemicals possess these antithyroid actions, but also a very large number of synthetic chemicals used on our foods and in our environment appear to damage the thyroid to different degrees.[28] So the more synthetic chemicals we are exposed to, the more our thyroid hormones are damaged and the fatter we will become.

STEROIDS

Many people already know that certain steroids used in medicine can add pounds. They include those that act on the sex hormones, such as the contraceptive pill. They also include steroids prescribed to prevent an asthma attack and some steroids used in cancer therapy. Side effects can make a patient blow up like a balloon and stimulate a ravenous appetite, particularly for carbohydrates.[29] So it is hardly surprising to learn that steroids have been used to fatten up animals for many years. In fact, some steroids are too good at increasing levels of body fat: When estrogens were given to broiler chickens, they caused such an increase in body fat that the practice had to be stopped; the meat was just too fatty to sell.[30]

More recently, because of food safety concerns, the use of steroids has been banned in animal farming across Europe, although they are still widely used in the United States.

You don't even have to be exposed to the steroids themselves to be affected, as a whole range of synthetic chemicals to which we are all commonly exposed can alter our natural levels of steroid hormones to induce the same fattening effects.[31]

The really scary thing about these steroids is that if they are given to pregnant animals, the offspring not only weigh more but also have higher weight gains all through their lives due to increased appetite and improved feed efficiency.[32]

ANTIBIOTICS

Antibiotics tend to have a more positive image because of their ability to clear up infections and kill germs. So when I found that antibiotics were commonly used to fatten animals, I assumed it was because they killed nasty bugs that made the animals lose weight through illness. What I didn't know then, but have discovered since, is that antibiotics will treat infections if given in high doses but not at the minute doses at which they are given to animals. However, they are present at a level that can promote animal weight gain.[33] Again, these chemicals appear to promote weight gain by damaging the weight control hormones and metabolism in such a way as to cause weight gain. Is this beginning to sound familiar?

The scale at which these antibiotics are used in animals is stunning. They account for more than half of the antibacterial drugs manufactured in the United States, and the vast majority of livestock will be exposed to antibacterial substances at some stage of their lives. Residues from antibiotics are found in meat from treated animals, so you will be taking them too and more often than you think. And although many antibiotics are naturally derived substances, an awful lot more are synthetic chemicals with the ability to fatten.[34]

But don't let this put you off taking a course of antibiotics if you need them. They can be life-saving, and the short, high-dose courses prescribed by doctors should not have a weight gain effect.

So, to sum up, all these chemicals are in the food chain today and have been there for a long time. Not only do they cause increased weight gain, but many have actually been formulated for that purpose. Considering our constant exposure to all these substances, just think what effect they're having on us. Is it any wonder we are in the grip of a fat epidemic?

The Human Growth Promoters

While the fact that synthetic chemicals make animals fat is of vital importance, the ultimate proof that these chemicals can make us fat is that doctors use them in hospital conditions for that very purpose.[35] It is obvious that if a drug is used deliberately to cause weight gain under medical supervision, a similar chemical will produce a similar effect if you are exposed to it from another source without realizing it.

I think that if people were more widely aware of the fact that, through pesticides in their food and pollutants in their environment, they are being exposed to chemicals similar to those used by doctors to fatten up patients, they wouldn't be too happy. So what are these substances, and how are we exposed to them?

There are quite a few medical conditions that cause people to lose too much weight. Anorexia is one obvious example. In the past, a large number of different "fattening" drugs have been used in an attempt to promote weight gain. Although this way of treating anorexia has been frowned upon recently, many drugs did appear to produce positive weight gain.[36]

One of these substances is sulpiride, a chemical that works by attacking and lowering the levels of our most powerful natural slimming hormones, our catecholamines. Indeed it is so powerfully fattening that if animals are exposed to it, they become obese within a short time. It is also a very commonly used antipsychotic medicine in psychiatry, which not so surprisingly causes great problems with unwanted weight gain during treatment. Because of these powerful fattening "side effects" and the ability to stabilize mental conditions, it has previously been tested to see whether it could be actively used to promote weight gain in anorexics.[37]

But we don't have to be on medication to get a dose of these chemicals, because we are exposed to a whole range of other catecholamine-attacking chemicals with actions very similar to those of sulpiride in our foods, again in the form of pesticide residues.

Elderly people can often suffer from a dramatic drop in weight due to loss of appetite. Drugs that have been used successfully to bring their weight back up again include corticosteroids and megestrol.[38] These and similar drugs were found to cause excessive weight gain when used to treat patients with breast and prostate cancer. Again, these substances are closely related to and have actions similar to certain pesticides used in our food.

A third group of people, cancer patients, are regularly treated with drugs to counteract the loss of appetite caused by cancer therapy. I have found a study that tested the ability of a bisthiocarbamate (see page 34) to prevent the normal dramatic fall in weight after toxic cancer therapy. In fact, it was so effective that it even produced mild weight gain.[39] The exact same chemical is one of the most common antifungal pesticides used in food production and is present in many fresh fruits and vegetables.

Weight Gain as a Known Side Effect

The other main way to show that synthetic chemicals have a fattening effect on humans is to look at the wealth of studies on the side effects of different medications. Everyone at some time in his or her life has known or heard of people who have had weight problems caused by a prescribed medication. The pill is one; steroids are another. In fact, a very large number of medications made up of synthetic chemicals can upset your metabolism, including some antihistamines, antinausea medications, a whole range of cardiovascular drugs, antifungals, certain antibiotics, and drugs to treat disorders of the nervous system.[40] Many of these, in particular medications used for the long-term treatment of illness, can also make you gain weight.

You will be horrified to find that you don't have to be on medication to be exposed to these compounds. Once again, very similar chemicals are found as pesticides in our foods or as pollutants in our environment.

But please understand that I'm not suggesting for one moment that you should stop taking medication if you are ill. The point I am making in all this is that there is abundant evidence that synthetic chemicals have the ability to make us fat. Moreover, we are being exposed to similar substances in our food and many nonfood products that could be making us fatter but without our knowledge or consent.

The Organochlorines You Have Accumulated Throughout Your Life Can Make You Fat

So now we know that there are a huge number of chemicals in our diet and environment that appear to cause weight gain. But how do we know that they are present at a level that will make us fat? Experts have estimated that each of us has on average approximately 300 to 500 industrial chemicals in our bodies, but it would be impractical and far too expensive to measure all of these routinely.[41]

The strongest evidence to show that we are contaminated with certain chemicals, at levels that appear to be making us fat, comes mainly from a group of extremely toxic pesticides and environmental pollutants more commonly known as organochlorines. Of the synthetic chemicals that we are now exposed to, organochlorines are possibly the most fattening of all. This is largely due to their ability to cause continual damage to our weight control systems, in combination with our relative inability to process them or get rid of them from our bodies.

Better-known members of this group are the extremely poisonous insecticides DDT and lindane, as well as a very common group of environmental pollutants known as polychlorinated biphenyls (PCBs). PCBs were once very widely produced and were used as fire retardants and insulating substances, but they have now been banned because of their extreme toxicity and longevity.

Despite many, but certainly not all, organochlorines having been banned for many years, they are still present in our bodies at levels far above those needed to damage our hormones, as unfortunately they tend to persist in our tissues for many decades.[42] They are also highly fat-soluble and tend to concentrate in fatty tissues. Because of these characteristics they are now present in most life forms, including humans. Since our bodies are virtually unable to break them up and kick them out, as the years go by, our stockpile of them just continues increasing.[43]

DDT, one of the most fattening of all the organochlorines, is one that has actually been banned for several decades in most developed countries but is still commonly found in people's bodies. Low levels of DDT have been shown to be powerful inducers of weight gain in animals.[44]

Lindane appears to be extremely fattening and has been shown to promote obesity in animals.[45] Despite being banned in at least eighteen countries and having its use severely restricted in ten others, it is still legal in the United States, where it is available in the form of flea sprays, insecticides, lawn treatments, and antilice shampoo. However, its use as an antilice shampoo is in the process of being banned in California. It is also present in many of our foods, particularly animal products.[46]

Yet another member of this fattening group is the pesticide hexachlorobenzene (HCB). As a pesticide it is widely banned, but large quantities of HCB continue to be produced and released into the environment as a waste by-product or impurity in the manufacture of pesticides and certain synthetic materials. Because of this and its longevity, it is still being found in the United States in a range of different foods, again mainly in animal products.[47] This organochlorine was found to possess such extreme fattening effects that in one animal study, when the food intake was cut by 50 percent, animals treated with HCB still managed to gain more weight than the untreated animals did on full rations![48]

Now this is where it gets kind of up close and personal. I have compared the levels of these organochlorines already present in our bodies with the levels that have been shown to cause weight gain in animals, and they are frighteningly similar. This suggests that our bodies are probably already being exposed to high enough levels of these organochlorines to make us gain weight. Despite the relative scarcity of scientific studies comparing organochlorine contamination and body weight, I managed to hit the jackpot with the few that I did uncover. These findings suggest that far from being just a hypothesis, the link between bodily contamination and excess weight appears to be very real. As with many of the previous studies, despite evidence suggesting that the greater the contamination by organochlorines, the greater the body weight, this vital connection was far from clear to the scientists performing the studies—probably because they were not looking for it.

Medical Studies Link Current Levels of Contamination to Increased Body Weight

A study carried out in Long Island, New York, looked at a number of ordinary women who did not have any reason to be exposed to dangerous chemicals at work or at home, or to eat foods from a known contaminated source. It revealed that those with higher levels of organochlorines in their bodies (measured in fat stores and circulating in their blood) generally had a higher body mass index (BMI); in other words, they were fatter than those who were less contaminated. By the way, the BMI is just a way of comparing your weight with your height to assess the level of body fat. Anyway, the study concluded that the accumulation of these contaminants over time was mainly due to the types of food these women ate.[49]

Several other studies provided further evidence that people who eat certain more contaminated foods were likely to be fatter. One study examined the effect of eating fish from the Great Lakes, which we know are relatively polluted with organochlorines (DDT and PCBs). It looked at fishermen who ate the salmon and trout that they caught from the lakes (as commercial fishing is banned, these were sport fishermen). Compared to the fishermen who didn't eat the fish they caught, the fish eaters had higher levels of PCBs and DDT as well as the heavy metals cadmium and lead. Significantly, they were also fatter.[50]

So, in summary, we now have real evidence to suggest that the level of contamination of the food we eat appears to affect our overall body weight. This is actually very positive, because if we can identify the foods that are more contaminated and therefore "fattening," we are well on the way to reducing our exposure to them in our diet.

So Why Aren't We All Fat?

If we gain weight by absorbing dangerous chemicals, and if these chemicals are all around us, then why aren't we all fat? We know from personal experience that many slim people eat sprayed and treated foods. The answer is most likely because of the differences in our genetic makeup and the many differences in our individual environments.

Beginning with the genetic differences, we know that some of us are born with detoxification systems that can detoxify and remove toxic substances better than can others. For example, approximately one-half of all Japanese individuals are born with an inherited inability to break down alcohol because of a lack of a certain detoxifying enzyme.[51] And this is only one of the many enzymes that needs to be working properly for us to be able to break down unwanted chemicals.

But it is not just our genes that make us all different. A whole number of other factors do too, such as our age;[52] our eating habits,[53] since certain foods tend to be more contaminated than do others; the level of nutrients we get in our diet, because a diet low in nutrients will prevent our detoxification systems from doing its job properly;[54] and finally the amount of chemical exposure we get from our environment.[55]

With so many factors involved, you can see it is not surprising that people vary greatly in their ability to detoxify and thereby maintain their weight.

Why Some Races Could Be More Prone to Weight Problems

It is not the least bit surprising, given all these factors, that there are differences among people within the same cultures as well as among those from different cultures in the ability to detoxify and control weight. It is the differences between races that could also account for why certain races tend to be more prone to weight gain than are others.[56]

For instance, Dr. Joellen Schildkrant from Duke University Medical Center found in a sample population of black and white women from North Carolina that black women had higher levels of organochlorines in their bodies than did white women. She also found that regardless of race, the higher the levels of chemicals, the heavier the woman would be. It is this mixture of genetic and cultural factors that could be at the bottom of why some races tend to have more weight problems than others.

Fortunately, the vast majority of the damage done by these chemicals is not permanent, and if you follow the advice given in the rest of this book, you will find out how to lose weight in such a way that it is extremely likely to stay off for good.

In the next chapter I will introduce the idea that we all have a highly developed weight control system, explain the way it works, and tell you what you need to do to maximize your ability to lose weight permanently. Please believe this: It is never too late to start. The fattening effects of chemicals really can be reversed. The secret of how to do it is here in these pages, so keep reading!

Your Natural *Slimming System:*
All About Your Highly Evolved
Weight Control System

This chapter is a vital one, because it lays the foundation for a fuller understanding of how chemicals can actually make us fat. Since you can only deal with a problem once you know what the problem is, the following pages will give you a unique insight into how the body controls its weight.

It cannot be denied that this is one of the more in-depth chapters, designed to give you a basic and thorough understanding of a whole range of essential dieting issues such as:

- What our natural *Slimming System* is and why it is so important.
- Why we have powerful food cravings and how to minimize them.
- How our body shape is controlled.
- Why dieting as we know it simply doesn't work.
- Why some people are more likely to gain weight than others.
- Why it can be extremely hard for some to lose excess body fat.
- The importance of the *Slimming System* in long-term weight control.
- Simple ways the *Slimming System* can be enhanced.

The chapter is packed with vital slimming information and advice to help you to maximize your weight loss. The bottom line is that by understanding how your body controls its weight, you will be able to see how this whole self-regulatory process has gone wrong. From there you will be able to work with your body, rather than against it, in order to put things right.

If however, you want to skip the theory part for now, you can go straight to Chapter 6 to discover "All About *Chemical Calories*" and come back to this and the following chapters at a later date.

We All Have a Natural *Slimming System*

In the battle of the bulge, our body has developed an extremely powerful weapon that can keep excess fat firmly at bay, if it is working well, but can result in us putting on weight if not. For want of a convenient term, I have dubbed this natural weight loss mechanism our *Slimming System*.

Our *Slimming System* covers a whole network of body systems, such as appetite, metabolism, hormone levels, fat burning, body heat, exercise, and more, which work together to maintain our ideal weight. Most experts agree that we all have an ideal weight and that our bodies will try to maintain it come famine or times of plenty by altering different parts of these weight control mechanisms. As most of these adjustments take place without us even knowing, we actually have much less direct control over our weight than we might imagine.

Just as our bodies have homeostatic mechanisms to maintain body temperature at a certain level, so too is our weight controlled by homeostatic mechanisms to maintain a largely predetermined weight "set point." This is the weight at which the body will try to remain.[1] In fact it can only be altered and set at a higher body weight if the underlying mechanisms get damaged.[2]

The fact that the average woman eats more than twenty tons of food between the ages of twenty-five and sixty-five, yet tends to gain only a fraction of this weight in pounds over these years, shows that the mechanisms used to maintain the set point are extremely efficient. If it is protected and well cared for, the ability to control our own weight can actually be a natural *Slimming System*.

Why We Need an
Efficient *Slimming System*

A person who has an efficient *Slimming System* will find it very easy to maintain his or her body weight. On the other hand, people with a less effective *Slimming System* will lack the same ability to burn off excess calories. So, unhappily for them, less food will go much further.

But the natural *Slimming System* doesn't just control weight, it also determines our body shape. The amount of muscle we have, whether we have a flat belly or a potbelly, slim hips or full hips—all this is determined by our natural *Slimming System*. So we can see that our *Slimming System* plays a key role in determining not only our weight but also our shape.

The problem at the heart of the fat epidemic is that most people's *Slimming Systems* appear to be constantly underachieving. This is because they are under attack from toxic chemicals and are lacking the nutrients they need in order to work properly.

The good news is that by reducing our exposure to the most damaging, or "fattening," of these chemicals and by increasing our intake of "slimming" nutrients, it suddenly becomes possible to revitalize our *Slimming System*. Once this happens, it can then start working properly to actively reduce our weight. But before we can find out the best way to repair our *Slimming System*, we need to know more about what exactly it is and how it works.

What Makes Up Our *Slimming System*?

The body's personal *Slimming System* is largely made up of the following four parts:

1. A control center (in the brain).
2. A large number of different "slimming" hormones.
3. An intact body structure.
4. A good supply of nutrients.

These four parts of the *Slimming System* are highly interdependent, with changes in one affecting all the others. Together they form a sort of dynamic body metabolism. A problem in any one of these areas could seriously reduce our overall ability to lose weight.

When these four parts are working well together, they alter our appetite, energy levels, and metabolism in such a way that our weight is kept low with virtually no conscious effort on our part. Let's find out more about these four key areas.

1. *Control Center*

The brain is where all weight control really happens. Messages about how much fat is stored are relayed from the brain around the body by hormones, which then feed information back to the brain. This information is processed in the control center, known as the *hypothalamus,* which is deep inside the brain and acts as the body's pilot.[3] If the brain thinks the fat stores are too large, it will send directions for the body to burn the excess off. If the brain thinks there is not enough fat stored, it will send signals to drive you to find something to eat. At all times, the constant aim is to keep your body at its predetermined weight set point.

But it works both ways, as the set point is itself determined by the efficiency of the whole *Slimming System.* So if the system has all the nutrients it needs to function properly and is intact and working well, the set point will be at a low level and the person will be lean. If, however, the system is not working smoothly and there are shortages of nutrients or damaged body organs, the set point will be higher, resulting in a fatter body.

For example, if the hypothalamus is injured, huge fluctuations in weight can occur as people lose their natural ability to control their appetite. This can get so extreme that people who have tumors in the hypothalamus area can, if untreated, actually die from overeating.

2. *Hormones*

If our brain is the most important part of our *Slimming System,* our hormones must be a close second. Hormones are natural chemical molecules acting as internal messengers that carry information and instructions around the body, enabling one part to talk to another. Although only minuscule amounts of hormones are produced, they control virtually all the body's functions, including food intake, ability to exercise, metabolism, maintenance of body heat, growth, reproduction, and, of course, the control of body size, weight, shape, and how much fat we store.[4]

All the major hormones, for example, the catecholamines, thyroid hormone, insulin, growth hormone, steroids, leptin, and the sex hormones (estrogen and testosterone), play a vital role in our *Slimming System*. Out of all these hormones, the catecholamines, more commonly known as our "fight or flight" hormones, are possibly the most important "slimming" hormones because of their prime role in enhancing fat burning.[5] They are produced by the nerve cells of the sympathetic nervous system (SNS), which is the part of the brain that coordinates the burning and storing of fat. As well as being produced in the brain, they are also produced by certain nerve endings throughout the rest of the body. As you will discover, they play a vital role in explaining the weight problems we are now facing.

3. *Intact Body Structure*

An intact and efficient body structure is essential in allowing all these vital processes to take place. For example, to burn up foods by exercising, we need our muscles to be working properly. And for our muscles to work, our nerves must be intact so they can stimulate the relevant muscles!

4. *Nutrients*

Last, but by no means least, our natural *Slimming System* needs a whole range of different nutrients such as vitamins, minerals, carbohydrates, proteins, and essential fatty acids. These nutrients power, accelerate, and facilitate the millions of individual reactions taking place in the body and so govern the overall speed of metabolism. The faster our metabolism is, the more fat we will use up. So you can see that an efficient metabolism is vital in order to keep in shape.

Now we will move on to discover the ways in which our *Slimming System* works to alter our appetite, the amount of exercise we do, and even our metabolism to maintain our weight at its optimum weight set point.

Appetite and Your *Slimming System*:
Are You Really in Charge of How Much You Eat?

Of all the messages controlled by your *Slimming System,* the one you will be most aware of is your appetite. You may think that you are in control of how much you eat, but in reality your hormones call all the shots. They manipulate your appetite according to what they perceive your present needs to be.

In fact, your hormones can even dictate the type of food you choose to eat, the amount you eat, and when you eat throughout the day. Different hormones stimulate an appetite for different foods, and as their levels change throughout the day, they will drive you to seek out whatever your body needs at any particular time.[6] So when you open the fridge door and decide what to eat next, you are not making an impartial choice. Your hormones running through your brain will guide your hand, telling you what your *Slimming System* wants.

For example, have you ever wondered why carbohydrates, such as toast, cereals, and fruit, are among the most commonly eaten foods for breakfast? Well, this is because your body needs readily available energy to get it powered up after the night's fast. As carbohydrates are the foods most easily converted into energy, the body produces large amounts of steroid hormones first thing in the morning to increase the appetite for carbohydrates.

It is a simple way of making sure that you make the right food choices. The carbohydrates will kick-start your body into action and replenish the small existing carbohydrate stores in the muscles and liver, which are essential for ensuring that you have lots of energy all day long.

Later in the day, once your body gets going, your appetite for other food groups, such as fats and proteins, will increase. This is achieved by a changing balance of a whole number of different hormones.

What Drives Us to Eat More Fat?

Our appetite for fat, on the other hand, is largely driven by the *absence* of hormones, specifically catecholamines. People fortunate enough to produce large amounts of catecholamines will tend to be lean and eat less fatty foods, because catecholamines suppress appetite in general and the desire for fatty foods in particular. They are known as the "fight or flight" hormones because they are released in stressful situations—and, as you can imagine, eating is the last thing you want to do if you're being chased by a bull!

Catecholamines work by increasing activity in the sympathetic nervous system (SNS), and an increase in SNS activity will automatically suppress the appetite. High levels of catecholamines also cause people to eat less fat. So a person with an active SNS tends to be driven to eat not only less food but also less fatty food.

The effect is so powerful that for many years now the most effective slimming pills have mimicked the appetite-suppressing effects of catecholamines. There are two main kinds of these appetite suppressants. The early ones caused the release of a natural catecholamine, dopamine, from its stores in the brain. These drugs were widely known as amphetamines and are rarely used now because of their potential for abuse. They have been replaced by a group of similar drugs with fewer side effects.

The Sheer Power of Hunger

This tendency to seek out specific foods to supply a particular nutrient is especially marked in pregnancy and is known as *pica*. It can cause a very powerful urge to eat, for example, raw meat or apples. The body will do all it can to persuade the pregnant woman to seek out foods with high levels of whatever nutrients it needs.

The same kind of thing happens in premenstrual women. The body needs more of a protein known as *phenylethylamine,* and, as large amounts of this substance are found in chocolate, the brain produces a craving for chocolate.[7]

Since our bodies keep adjusting our appetite according to our needs, it makes extreme dieting (and, in particular, restrictive single-food diets) very difficult to follow. Your brain will deliberately do its very best to make you break the diet, increasing your appetite sharply to send you off in search of food.

Constant hunger pangs and food cravings are very uncomfortable to ig-

nore—precisely because your body has been designed to give in to them!
This obviously makes trying to control your weight simply by eating less
food very difficult to do, as you end up fighting your own drives and needs.[8]
This is why very restrictive diets are exceedingly uncomfortable and usually
fail in the long run.

How Body Shape Is Controlled
by the *Slimming System*

Not only does the *Slimming System* control weight, it also controls our basic
body shape. Several of the "slimming hormones" also play major roles here,
but two of the most important ones are the male and female sex hormones.

The male sex hormone, testosterone, builds muscle and burns fat,
causing men to be generally leaner and more muscular than women. A reduction in the levels of testosterone as men get older creates a tendency for
muscles to shrink and fat to gather, particularly around the abdominal area;
in other words, it is largely responsible for a paunch.[9]

The female sex hormones, estrogens, encourage fat storage, particularly
in the breasts, thighs, and buttocks. This is most obvious during puberty,
when rising levels of female sex hormones create the curvy outline we normally associate with women. It also explains why women tend to store more
body fat than do men and why women on the pill can sometimes gain weight.

Exercise and the *Slimming System*

Exercise is a vitally important tool in maintaining our weight. It is also one of
the few ways in which you can positively reduce your weight set point and
improve your body shape.[10] This is not just because exercise burns off lots
of calories, but because when you exercise you will actually increase your
body's production of certain vital "slimming" hormones.[11] This hormonal effect lasts way beyond short-term calorie burning, as after good spells of exercise these slimming effects can extend for several days or even weeks.

Once again, you might think that the amount of exercise you engage in is totally voluntary. In fact, your level of spontaneous activity is strongly controlled by your hormones and depends on an intact body structure and all the necessary nutrients that generate energy to power the muscles.

We all differ in our natural activity levels, even from birth. Some babies are far more active than others and will tend to grow up to be the type of people who seem to have endless energy, take part in more strenuous activities, and are constantly on the go.[12] These fortunate people are far less likely to have a weight problem than those born with a lower energy drive, who tend to exercise less, tire more easily, and have to make more of a conscious effort to exercise.

So what determines our energy drive? Well, our hormones do. Hormones affect both long-term and short-term aspects of muscle metabolism; they stimulate growth, maintain muscle volume, increase energy levels in muscle, and alter our metabolism to make available the foods necessary for sufficient levels of energy production. Though a wide range of hormones may play a role in controlling the amount of exercise we engage in, the catecholamines play the leading role. So you can see why they make such good slimming aids. They can reduce your appetite, but they can also increase your energy levels[13] so that you feel like engaging in more exercise throughout all aspects of your life.

Catecholamines not only increase your conscious activity, such as walking, but they also increase the amount of involuntary fidgeting movements you make.[14] Although you may not be so aware of them, these fidgeting actions can burn up quite a significant amount of energy and can play an important part in allowing your *Slimming System* to do its job.

What Reduces Our Ability to Exercise?

Although we inherit much of our body chemistry, which largely determines how active we are, several other factors also affect the amount of energy we produce. They include metabolic disorders, hormone imbalances, and even a lack of essential nutrients in the food that we eat.

Most people don't appreciate how our hormones stimulate the will to exercise until they have a hormone deficiency or imbalance. A feeling of fatigue or lack of energy is one of the most common symptoms of hormone problems and is also commonly found in people with vitamin or mineral deficiencies.

Moreover, damage to any part of the body structure involved in exercise, from the nerves stimulating the muscles to damaged muscle fibers, will prevent us from burning off calories through exercise. As the body uses up approximately 25 percent of the energy derived from food in exercise, a reduced ability to exercise resulting from damage or illness would most definitely affect the overall balance—increasing the chances of weight gain.

Why Our Energy Levels Can Fall Dramatically When Dieting

Just as your body alters your appetite to adapt to changing circumstances, so too is your body able to alter its energy levels to control the amount of exercise you take.

Fluctuating energy levels are particularly noticeable if you cut your food back in an attempt to lose weight. Because of the shortage of nutrients, rather than "wasting" them on powering nonessential exercise, the body will redirect them to power its most important life-support systems.

The resulting feelings of fatigue and lack of energy are therefore a natural defense mechanism to prevent you from doing too much under these conditions—your body effectively compensates by dropping your energy levels so that you exercise less. It will also cut your level of involuntary movement (fidgeting) to save even more energy.

This helps to explain why crash dieting rarely works, as the body instinctively tries to protect itself from a sudden weight loss by dramatically reducing the desire to exercise. And, if you force yourself to take exercise strenuously on a limited food intake, for the remainder of the day your body will tend to reduce the amount of energy you spend on nonessential tasks by dramatically reducing your energy levels—making you feel tired and forcing you to rest.

Weight control mechanisms also kick in if you try to lose weight by simply increasing your level of exercise. For example, if you spend thirty minutes every day doing vigorous aerobics, the extra exercise will definitely help you lose lots of excess fat and develop more body muscle. However, you will not burn off twenty-seven pounds of body fat after a year, which is the fat equivalent of the number of calories used up from the aerobic exercises. This is because your natural weight control mechanisms actively compensate to some extent for this higher activity level.

By the same token, if you change from a very active job to a less active one, your appetite will reduce to compensate.[15] This ability to compensate is known as your *dynamic metabolism*.

Your Metabolism and the *Slimming System*

Figure 4 shows how the body uses up the energy we get from the foods we eat.[16] You can see that exercise uses up only a quarter of your daily intake of food, while another quarter is burned off by hormones such as catecholamines. But clearly the biggest energy user of all is the body's basic metabolism. Since our metabolism is such a major player in weight control, it is important to understand what it is and how it works.

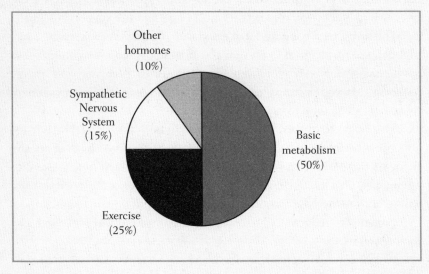

Figure 4. The relative importance of different systems in using up energy

Metabolism is a convenient term to cover the billions of reactions taking place in our bodies to convert food to fat or energy. On average, just keeping your vital functions running accounts for about half of the energy you burn off every day. The speed of metabolism, or *metabolic rate*, can vary quite a lot from person to person.[17] Two people can be exactly the same size and have the same amounts of muscle and fat, yet the person with the faster metabolism can burn up more calories. This means that the person with the slower metabolism has to eat less than does the person with the faster metabolism to stay at the same weight.

What determines whether you are a faster or slower fat burner? Well, surprise, surprise, your hormones do. Hormones, or the lack of them, strongly influence the speed of your metabolism. For example, an excess of thyroid hormone can actually double your metabolic rate, resulting in weight loss, whereas a deficiency can reduce it by more than half, causing weight gain. So the overall speed or efficiency at which our hormones are working will play a very important role in determining where our weight set point will be fixed.

What Underlies an Efficient Fat-Burning Metabolism?

Your hormones have a natural rhythm that helps to order the metabolic reactions in a way that maximizes the efficiency of the entire process. A deficiency in one particular hormone or nutrient can disrupt the overall rhythm, thereby reducing the efficiency of the reactions. In order to keep these processes working to full capacity, we need to ensure that we feed our metabolism with all the essential nutrients it needs to work as well as provide it with enough vitamins and minerals to act as catalysts for all the millions of reactions taking place.

I'll go into much more detail about nutrients and supplements to power your metabolism in Chapter 13: Repair and Revitalize Your Natural *Slimming System*. For now, the important thing is to realize that a good metabolic rate is vital if you want to keep your weight down.

How We Burn Off Excess Fat Stores

The hormones that control metabolism are also in control of the rate at which fat is burned up, and the most important hormones in this process are, once again, the catecholamines. They are vital to our ability to burn off body fat stores; without them, we simply could not break down fat.

Another way in which our body burns up large amounts of energy is in controlling our body temperature. The heat-producing process known as *thermogenesis* is designed to keep us warm if the temperature drops, but it also helps the body burn off excess food by raising the overall body temperature to a higher level than normal.[18] In this way, excess food or body fat stores can be converted into heat that can then be easily dispersed.

Carbohydrates in particular are good at increasing heat production. This helps to explain why you will get a warm feeling after eating foods rich in carbohydrates. Their ability to release catecholamines into the body ensures that excess carbohydrates are burned off and not stored as fats.

What Happens to Our Metabolism When We Diet?

Traditional methods of dieting depend on the idea that a certain amount of food has a fixed caloric value and that by cutting your food intake you will lose weight. However, the body's dynamic metabolism means that if you cut your intake of calories, your body will respond to this pretty quickly by slowing down the rate at which you burn off food as heat. In this way, your body can conserve internal energy. This has the effect of making less food go further.

This is a basic survival mechanism that protects (among others) pregnant or lactating women in poorer countries. Rather than starve the baby of food, the mother's body will shut down any waste of food energy. This mechanism is so powerful that even mothers with physically demanding jobs can produce adequate amounts of breast milk to feed their babies.[19]

Ideally, if your *Slimming System* is working well, the reverse will happen if you overeat. The rate at which your body produces heat should increase until you burn off all the excess food.

This dynamic metabolism explains why dieting by food restriction alone will never work in the long term. The body will strive to return to its set point not just when you are dieting but also after you stop. Dieting alone simply cannot alter the weight set point and only makes the body more efficient with the food it has got. So, while you can lose weight in the short term, when you stop dieting your body will do all it can to compensate for the food shortage, and you will end up weighing at least as much as you did before you started.

I think by now it should be absolutely clear that you will never be able to lose weight by following traditional dieting methods alone. The experience of the past fifty years or more backs this up completely. With such a large chunk of the population dieting at any one time, if traditional diets really worked there would actually be few fat people left!

Overweight People Have Less Effective Metabolisms

It will come as no surprise to any of you who are actually eating less than your slimmer friends that overweight people appear to have less efficient metabolisms. The same amount of food that will maintain the weight of slimmer people can make overweight people fatter. What's more unfair is that overweight people also appear to use up proportionately less energy in carrying out a whole range of different body functions.

Studies have shown that in overweight people there is a basic malfunctioning in the most important part of the body's *Slimming System*—the sympathetic nervous system (SNS).[20] People who have an underactive SNS will tend to have greater appetites, particularly for fatty foods, since they produce fewer fat-burning catecholamines. The amount of energy they appear to burn up to heat the body is likely to be lower.[21] They even seem to use up less energy than a naturally slimmer person would use if he or she engaged in the same amount of exercise.[22] This obviously creates an energy imbalance, as the number of calories taken in is far greater than the number being used up. These excess calories may then be stored as fat deposits.

Overweight People Are Also Less Able to Use Up Their Existing Fat Stores

But the problem doesn't stop there, because the SNS needs to be functioning properly for fats to be released from adipose tissue. As the SNS is less active, the total rate at which fat can be used up from these stores could plummet.

So, with less fat readily available to burn, overweight people tend to produce less heat after eating a meal or when their surroundings get colder. Since they cannot raise their body temperature as much as lean people, they use up less excess body fat and end up getting colder and fatter. So despite the ever-increasing stores of fat being there, they simply cannot actively mobilize them and use them up.

The bad news is that even if they do lose weight temporarily by traditional food-restriction diets, they will still have an underactive SNS, so the struggle to keep excess weight off will continue throughout their lives.

Now don't despair at this point. There *is* a way to boost your *Slimming System* and SNS to a new level of improved functioning that will lower your weight set point and therefore your body weight as well.

Many of the toxic chemicals we are regularly exposed to not only damage the *Slimming System* but also specifically target the SNS.[23] This damage could result in increasing the overall weight set point. By reducing our exposure to these chemicals, the *Slimming System* can be revived and allowed to function properly again.

Overweight People Are Low in Certain Vitamins and Minerals

There is one more vitally important difference between overweight and lean people: Compared to the non-overweight, overweight people tend to be markedly deficient in certain vitamins and minerals. Just because you are getting enough calories in your diet doesn't automatically mean that you are getting enough vitamins and minerals. On the contrary, the fatter you are, the more deficient you are likely to be.[24]

So it will hardly come as a surprise that the vitamins and nutrients that overweight people lack are the same ones that play vital roles in maximizing the ability to burn off fat.[25] This shortfall in vital nutrients not only reduces your ability to lose weight but also starts a vicious circle, making your whole system less efficient.

I know that if I forget to take my vitamins for more than one day, by the second evening I can really feel fatigue coming on. To me, this is a sign that my metabolism hasn't got what it needs to produce enough energy to power my body fully. If being tired makes you exercise less, then you have little chance of burning off excess food.

Which Nutrients Seem to Be Missing?

So which vitamins and minerals are we talking about? Well, in all the studies I have read, the ones cropping up again and again are vitamins A, B, C, and E, and the minerals zinc and magnesium. In fact, studies have shown that the fatter a person becomes, the more likely it is that he or she will be deficient in vitamins A, C, and E, and several of the B group vitamins.

In a study of very overweight women, 58 percent were deficient in vitamin C, but among women of average weight the deficiency level was a very low 3 percent.[26] In another important study carried out by the U.S. government (National Health and Nutritional Examination Survey III [NHANESIII]), Dr. Strauss compared the concentration of vitamins E and A in obese and nonobese American children and found that obese children were far more likely to have significantly lower blood levels of vitamins A and E than were normal weight children.[27]

The evidence that these vitamins play a crucial part in our *Slimming System* was supported by yet another study that found that if obese nondieting women were given 1 gram of vitamin C three times a day for a period of six weeks, they lost 5.5 pounds without even trying to diet.[28]

This is potentially very good news, because it suggests that, for whatever reason, overweight people tend to be extremely deficient in certain nutrients that are vital to the smooth running of their *Slimming Systems*. It opens up the possibility that one of the reasons overweight people *are* over-weight is because they lack the appropriate nutrients to bring about weight loss, either because they use up nutrients faster than the average person or because their diet is particularly lacking in them, or a combination of both factors.

This problem is actually much more common than you might suspect. The number of people worldwide thought to be deficient in at least one vi-tamin or mineral has been estimated at a stunning 2 to 3.5 billion—many of these being people who are overweight.[29] Taking the appropriate vitamin supplements allows the *Slimming System* to function properly, perhaps for the first time ever, and so works to burn off excess weight and keep it off.

It also appears that deficiencies in certain vitamins and minerals could be partly responsible for altering body shape. The evidence is strongest for vitamin E. For example, a study by Ohrvall in 1993 found that the lower the level of vitamin E in the blood, the greater the abdominal measurement.[30]

In another study, researchers looked at Indian men with abdominal obesity. It found that the more abdominal fat they had, the lower their blood levels of vitamin E, vitamin C, magnesium, and zinc.[31] Again, this is actu-ally marvelous news, as it is relatively easy to remedy vitamin and mineral deficiencies by taking the right balance of supplements.

To optimize your *Slimming System*, it is now clear that you need to give your body all the nutrients it needs to work to its maximum ability (see Chapter 15).

Use Your Natural *Slimming System*

The aim of this chapter has been to show you that willpower alone is not your greatest asset in losing weight. Your greatest asset is, in fact, a healthy and efficient *Slimming System*, as any attempt to lose weight by just reduc-ing the amount of food you eat will be countered by the body doing all it can to fight the change. It will increase your appetite, reduce the amount of ex-ercise you do, and even reduce the rate at which you burn off calories. Your body will maintain its existing food stores as if its life depended on it—mil-lions of years ago, it probably did!

The only effective way forward for those of you who want to lose weight permanently is to get your body to work with you in losing weight rather than fighting against you all the way.

This next chapter will explain how chemicals have poisoned the body's natural *Slimming System*. This totally new and groundbreaking information has never previously been published in a book and will completely change our approach to weight loss. By understanding just how these chemicals damage us, we move one step closer not only to preventing any further damage but also to restoring our *Slimming System* to its former glory.

5

How Chemicals Make You Fat:
Why Dieting Without
Detox Will Fail

You may not have realized it, but there is a war going on inside your body. As you read this, synthetic chemicals are currently engaged in an increasingly one-sided battle against your natural *Slimming System.* Judging by the number of overweight people, the chemicals appear to be winning hands down.

The evidence that many of these highly toxic substances have the ability to destroy our natural weight control systems is overwhelming. What's more, it seems that this is happening at our current exposure levels. In order to win the battle against chemicals, and win it we most definitely can, we need to raise our defenses and fortify our shields. This, in a nutshell, is what this chapter is all about.

It will tell you how toxic chemicals are able to attack every single major part of our *Slimming System,* how the subsequent damage can make us fat, the ways in which chemicals can alter our body shape, how traditional methods of dieting can make us fatter, and, last but not least, how the fundamental way in which we diet has to change in order to adapt to the new environment in which we find ourselves.

Like the previous chapter, it will be more detailed than the rest of the book, but the proof of the pudding is in the eating, so to speak, and I think that after you have read it you will understand why I have spent so much time clarifying these issues.

So take heart: Weight gain is not simply due to weak willpower, gluttony, and laziness. Most of it is due to your body's inability to deal with toxins in your food and environment. And once you understand exactly what is happening, you will be well on your way toward dealing with the problem. Please believe me when I say that there is light at the end of the tunnel, because by reading this book you will be brought yet another step closer to achieving the body of your dreams. Go on—you're worth it!

What Makes Our *Slimming System* One Of The First Systems "Hit" by These Well-Armed Invaders?

Toxic chemicals are well known for their ability to damage a whole number of body systems. However, there are certain reasons why our *Slimming System* is probably more susceptible to chemical damage than the rest of our other body systems.

The most important tissues making up our *Slimming System,* for example, our brain, glands, and body fat, tend to have a high fat content and a relatively good blood supply. Unfortunately, tissues that have these characteristics tend to be more vulnerable to chemical damage. The first problem relates to the fact that many of the more toxic synthetic chemicals are extremely fat soluble. So when they are released into the blood, they make a beeline for the fattier parts of the body. Due to their high fat content, the most central parts of the *Slimming System* present an easy target for these chemicals.

Second, as the brain and our hormone-secreting glands have some of the largest blood supplies of all the existing organs in our body, they end up being exposed to the largest amounts of blood-borne toxins.[1]

As a result, the most toxic and persistent synthetic chemicals tend to concentrate in the most sensitive and vulnerable parts of our *Slimming Sys-*

tem. So it comes as no surprise that out of all the systems in our body, our *Slimming System* will be among the first in line to be damaged by chemicals.

Now that we know what makes our *Slimming System* particularly vulnerable to injury, we need to move on to discover exactly what kind of damage takes place. Let's return to the four main parts of our *Slimming System* and see how this fattening effect is brought about in each individual situation.

Brain and Nerve Damage

The brain controls everything about who we are and what we do. No exception is made when it comes to body weight and eating, as the brain governs all our eating behavior, appetite, and metabolism. On top of this, it also controls the body's weight set point.

Unfortunately, the brain is exquisitely sensitive to damage from all kinds of chemical toxins, not only because of its high fat content and excellent blood supply but also because it appears to be less able than most parts of the body to deal with certain chemical toxins.[2] In addition, unlike most other tissue, once poisoned, many brain cells cannot regenerate themselves.

Here is an example of how our brain is put at risk by these chemicals. One of the features that makes certain synthetic chemicals "good" pesticides is their ability to act as nerve agents, paralyzing the functioning of certain parts of the brain.[3] The probability is high that many of the pesticides in our food will act on us in a way similar to the way they act on insects. To put it brutally, many of the chemicals deliberately added to our food could therefore be acting as small doses of nerve agent on our brains. How does that grab you?

Hormones, the Fat Controllers

When I was in the midst of my research, it didn't take long before I realized that virtually every one of the pesticides found in our foods—in addition to the majority of the other synthetic chemicals I was investigating—appeared to have a significant effect on at least one of the major weight-controlling hormones. More specifically, the trend was that these chemicals tended to increase the levels of fattening hormones, such as insulin and steroids,[4] while reducing the levels of slimming hormones, such as thyroid hormone, sex hormones, growth hormone, and catecholamines.[5]

Our Natural "Slimming" Hormones, Catecholamines, Are Targeted

It appeared to me during the course of my research that out of all the hormones affected by chemicals, those that seemed to come most frequently under attack were our most valuable group of slimming hormones, the catecholamines. Not only was a powerful catecholamine-lowering effect evident in animals, but it was also frequently found in humans.

For example, one study of workers in a pesticide factory manufacturing organochlorines, organophosphates, and carbamates revealed that the workers themselves produced at least 40 percent fewer "slimming" catecholamines in their blood than the average person.[6]

This may be explained in part by the fact that the adrenal gland, which is responsible for producing a large amount of "slimming" catecholamines, has been described as the gland most susceptible to chemical-induced toxicities.[7] With fewer catecholamines being produced, is it any wonder that we are losing the ability to stay slim?

Body Structure

To burn off excess food, the basic fabric of your whole body needs to be in good shape. The problem is that many chemicals can directly injure much of our body's basic structure. As many of these chemicals can also inhibit the amount of body protein created, the overall structural damage is magnified.

As protein-rich structures make up much of our body structure and in particular much of the fabric of our *Slimming System* (specifically in the form of hormones, enzymes, mitochondria, and muscles), chemical damage has a dramatic domino effect on the entire efficiency of our *Slimming System*.

A good example of this effect is provided by sheep farmers. Those who dip their sheep in organophosphate sheep dips to kill parasites were found to have smaller calf muscles than quarry workers who do a similar amount of work but have no contact with organophosphates.[8] This well-documented muscle-shrinking effect is thought to be caused in the following way. First, the nerves that stimulate the muscles are damaged or destroyed, and the muscle they would normally stimulate ends up just wasting away. Second, the muscle fibers themselves as well as the energy-producing mitochondria that exist within the muscle can be directly damaged by these chemicals, which promotes muscle shrinkage and a lower level of energy production.[9]

In addition to shrinking muscles, the level of stamina is diminished as muscles become fatigued more quickly. This is a direct result of a slowdown in energy production, such that the supply can no longer meet the demand. This is why the most common symptoms of chemical toxicity are weak muscles and general fatigue.[10] You can imagine that if you don't feel like exercising, you are far less likely to burn off excess body fat. If marked, this muscle toxicity can make you feel so tired that you don't want to get out of bed, let alone go for a walk.

Synthetic Chemicals Are Depleting Your Body of Its "Slimming" Nutrients

To ensure the smooth running of the body's natural *Slimming System*, we need to provide it with all the fuel it needs and cannot manufacture itself, such as vitamins, minerals, proteins, and certain essential fats. A shortage of any one of these vital nutrients may seriously reduce the overall efficiency of your entire *Slimming System*.

Synthetic chemicals have had a major destructive role even here. It seems that not only can they interfere with the way our bodies absorb nutrients from foods, but they also can directly destroy some of the more delicate nutrients, prevent the production of other essential nutrients, increase the rate at which the body uses various nutrients, and even increase the rate at which the body excretes nutrients.[11]

So the overall effect is to promote in our bodies a form of chemically induced nutrient deficiency that involves all the previously mentioned nutrients but perhaps most of all the antioxidants, namely vitamins C and E. This is because when toxic chemicals damage our tissues, the body needs to repair the harm caused by the subsequent blast of free radicals released. As the body soaks up free radicals with antioxidants, this could explain why our need for these particular vitamins seems to have skyrocketed.[12] In addition, these chemicals appear to deprive our *Slimming System* of a whole range of nutrients essential for its smooth functioning. And if the *Slimming System* cannot work to its full capacity, chances are we will end up gaining weight.

Our Need for Certain Nutrients Has Been Permanently Increased

Because of the increasing presence of synthetic chemicals in our bodies and lives, our need for certain nutrients has increased to a level greater than it has probably ever been. We now appear to need doses of certain nutrients far higher than those commonly laid down as guidelines, because these values were simply not created with chemical damage in mind.

Regrettably, our nutrient intake from food has in all likelihood dropped to an all-time low. To aggravate an already bad situation, we are now deriving a fraction of the nutrients that we once did thousands of years ago. The problem is that even by eating the perfect diet of nutrient-rich foods, our need for certain vitamins has increased so much that we will never be able to get the levels we need from our food alone—even with the best will in the world.[13]

Fortunately, this situation can be fully dealt with. By taking the right supplements, you can give your body the nutrients it needs to power its vital systems as well as its *Slimming System* and, in so doing, help combat any potential damage by chemicals. The recommended doses of nutrients are given in Chapter 15.

How Chemicals Can Increase Your Appetite

As we have seen in the previous chapter, hormones control our appetite. So it is not surprising to discover that hormone-damaging toxic chemicals can also have a powerful influence on our appetite.[14] What tends to happen is that chemicals can disturb the usually precise balance between the amount of food we eat and the amount of food we actually require. The overall effect is an increased appetite that can drive us to eat more than our body actually needs.

This appetite-enhancing effect is one of the more important ways that synthetic chemicals can work in promoting animal growth and is a major reason for the effectiveness of many chemicals that have been used to fatten up humans. It also appears to contribute to the powerful fattening side effects of certain medications such as steroids and antihistamines.[15] Ask anyone on even a short course of steroids, and they will tell you how their cravings for carbohydrates escalated.

However, not only is our overall level of appetite affected, but the hormones damaged are those that control our appetite for fatty and sugary foods, the catecholamines and steroids, so that if the level of these hormones is altered, our desire for these foods can increase. Perhaps this explains the popularity of fast foods, since they meet the criteria of increased fats and sugars perfectly. Unless we can fight our body's natural urges every day, chemical damage could make us eat more than we need. And I don't imagine for one second that you need me to tell you that this will ultimately make us fatter.

Chemical Damage and a
Reduced Ability to Exercise

Yet again, synthetic chemical interference appears to severely affect all aspects of our ability to exercise, making our get-up-and-go simply dwindle. I must admit that when I started researching the effects these chemicals have on our ability to exercise, I never anticipated finding such wide-ranging and damaging results, as all aspects of muscle function seem to be touched.

As well as shrinking the muscles, which reduces strength and stamina, they also reduce our energy drive. And at this point, the catecholamines come into the equation again. Besides controlling our appetite, they also effectively "set" our energy levels and our desire to exercise. Consequently, any fall in catecholamine levels, such as the reductions produced by an extremely large number of synthetic chemicals, not only will reduce the amount of voluntary exercise we feel like engaging in, but also will probably lessen the involuntary movements that we usually don't even notice.[16] The overall effect is rather like a chemical sledgehammer.

Adding further insult to injury, chemically damaged muscles will probably be less able than nondamaged muscles to burn up energy.[17] This will reduce our ability to burn up calories even further. This damage to our ability to exercise will have a serious effect on our overall weight, as exercise is one of the main ways in which our bodies burn off excess calories.

Again, don't despair as you read this. It is possible to regain your natural energy drive, even if it is currently low. By following the instructions in this book, you can overcome this chemical damage to improve not only your natural energy levels but also your level of fitness. Just keep reading and soon all will be revealed!

How Chemical Damage Affects Metabolism

The last major part of our *Slimming System* to be considered is our metabolism. As our basic metabolism is by far the biggest user of energy, any damage to our metabolism, however small, can have very serious weight implications.

Once again, synthetic chemicals can damage virtually all aspects of our metabolism. By lowering the amount of hormones that speed up metabolism and by reducing the availability of a whole range of essential nutrients—by using them up to rid the body of these new chemicals—they can effectively slow down the rate of energy production.[18] This ability to reduce energy expenditure means that they make great animal fatteners, since less food goes further. But, on the other hand, they can devastate our ability to lose weight or to stay slim.

In addition, as if we needed more bad news, our ability to use up certain foods—for example, carbohydrates—also appears to be impaired by certain chemicals.[19] This could be one of the reasons a diet high in carbohydrates leads so easily to weight gain.

But, despite this apparent slowdown, we still need a certain amount of carbohydrates in our diet, because they powerfully rev up our metabolism by stimulating the production of catecholamines. They are also essential to our ability to detoxify chemicals.[20] So eating carbohydrates in moderation, rather than cutting them out completely, seems to be the answer.

Chemicals Prevent Us from Using Up Our Fat Stores

But it is not only carbohydrates that are affected. Synthetic chemicals specifically appear to reduce our ability to burn up our existing fat stores.[21] This is probably done in two main ways: first, by lowering our ability to generate body heat,[22] and second, by reducing the levels of hormones essential for releasing body fats from storage.[23]

Chemical damage appears to make people less able to raise their body temperature—an effect that is particularly apparent when surrounding temperatures fall. This can be seen in people who are severely damaged by chemicals, as they tend to have a lower-than-average body temperature.[24] So if they produce less heat, they end up using less energy.

The reason for this inability to convert existing fat stores into heat is that the hormones that are essential in mobilizing fats, namely catecholamines, have been severely lowered. Because of this, our fat stores cannot be exploited fully to produce heat energy or indeed energy for any other reason. So, once our fat is in storage, it becomes very difficult to shift, creating ever-increasing amounts of fat stores that our bodies simply cannot use up.

Weight control, then, is not just a matter of regulating what we eat and how much we exercise; it also involves a huge diversity of systems that can all be damaged by chemicals. You can see for yourself that your weight depends far less on your willpower than on the state of your *Slimming System*.

Not Just Heavier, But Fatter Too

Yet more bad news: Not only do toxic chemicals appear to make us heavier, but some of these chemicals could also make us fatter. As the pounds pile up, certain chemicals tend to increase the proportion of body fat while simultaneously lowering the proportion of body muscle.[25] The overall result is a fatter, less shapely body.

And it doesn't stop there: These changes could have an add-on effect on our skin too. As there is a certain amount of muscle in skin, any subsequent reduction in the amount of muscle will affect the firmness of the skin, making it softer and flabbier.

In addition to worsening the condition and appearance of our skin, these chemicals could also increase our amount of cellulite. This is because the packages of fat stored under the skin will be held in less firmly and will be more visible if the skin is thinner.

Why Certain Families Seem to Have More Weight Problems Than Others

You might ask, "Since we are all exposed to these chemicals, why aren't we all fat?" After all, most slim people eat contaminated foods and live in the same environment. The answer is related to the overall amount of pollutants that we are exposed to and to our nutritional status, as well as to our individual ability to deal with toxins.

For years, the view was that people were stuck with the particular balance of hormones that they were born with. The ability to inherit "overweight" genes was thought to explain why the problem of excess weight tended to run in families and left people believing that there was absolutely nothing they could do about their weight if they inherited these genes.

Now it is clear that our body chemistry can be totally altered by toxic chemicals. So perhaps what these families have really inherited is a vulnerability to toxic chemical damage. We already know that there is a huge genetically based variation in our ability to detoxify certain chemicals.[26] For instance, some racial groups cannot metabolize alcohol as well as others.

In addition to explaining why some racial groups seem to be vastly more susceptible to weight gain than others, this raises the possibility that people from fatter families could now become thinner by reducing their exposure to toxic chemicals and by eliminating their body stores of fattening chemicals.

Why Is the Epidemic Growing So Fast?

If you turn back to Figure 1, you will see that this fat epidemic is a relatively recent problem. The big question is: Why is the epidemic growing at such a rapid pace? The most obvious reason by far is the ever-increasing level of chemicals to which we are now exposed. However, before we can deal with the problem effectively, a full understanding of the possible reasons is essential. By looking at the broader picture, several other likely reasons emerge: these increasing chemical stores we gather throughout our lives, our worsening nutrition, and our increased tendency to diet.

Why We Are Becoming Increasingly Fatter as We Get Older

It is a sad fact that adults are gaining weight throughout their lives at a greater speed than ever before. This increasing tendency to gain weight as we get older can largely be ascribed to several different factors. First, throughout our lives our body load of chemicals tends to increase. The greater the buildup, the more disrupted the *Slimming System* will be. Second, these increased levels of chemicals will most probably result in a greater level of existing *Slimming System* damage. And last, the body's detoxification system also tends to become less effective as we get older.[27]

How Our Increasingly Processed Foods and Nutrient-Poor Diets Make Us Fatter

Given the quantity of toxic chemicals in our food and environment and the way they increase our need for nutrients, it has been said that even the most well-balanced diet could not contain all the nutrients we now need without some form of supplementation.[28] Food processing, storage, and conventional farming techniques have all done their bit to reduce the quality of protein, vitamins, and minerals now present in our food. Add to this the fact that an extremely large percentage of the population is now actively dieting, and this reduces the chances of getting sufficient nutrients from food even further.

So, on the one hand, our need for nutrients has actually grown, but on the other, our *Slimming Systems* are being increasingly starved of the nutrients they need. Not surprising, the consequences of this increasing nutrient imbalance are now clearly evident in our escalating weight problem.

How Conventional Dieting Can Actually Make Us Fatter

While you may think you are doing the right thing by going on a conventional diet, you could actually make your weight problem worse. This is because when you diet, your body will have to burn up more fat to power its systems.

You might think this is a good thing, and it probably was hundreds of years ago. However, your fat stores now contain a large amount of accumulated toxic chemicals, which are mobilized into your system in a big *whoosh* as soon as you start burning off your fat.[29] Once set free in your body, these toxins will redistribute themselves and cause havoc in the most vulnerable parts of your *Slimming System*.

Then there is also the problem of insufficient nutrients, because by restricting your intake of food, you will have fewer nutrients to repair the damage.

So every time you go on a diet without protecting your body against the release of stored toxins and chemicals, you will be effectively damaging your *Slimming System*. This is most probably why people who lose weight quickly seem to put back the weight they have lost, plus a bit extra. This can also explain why the next time you try to diet, it seems even harder, because in truth it really will be.

Yet, if done in the right way, you can use food-restriction dieting to lose weight. However, here the whole method has to be changed. Rather than using food-restriction alone, the emphasis is on detoxification and on protecting your natural *Slimming System*. The upside is potentially fantastic though, for if done properly, not only can *Chemical Calorie* detox dieting accelerate your eventual weight loss, but it can also lower your body weight set point.

How Do You Know if Your *Slimming System* Is Damaged?

There has been a lot of talk about what causes damage to the *Slimming System*, but how do we actually know if our *Slimming System* is damaged?

Well, the biggest and most obvious sign that your *Slimming System* is flagging is if you are already overweight. Another sign is easy weight gain, especially if it seems a daily struggle to keep your weight down.

Other relevant clues include a great desire to eat fatty and sugary foods, a tendency to feel the cold, and a changing body shape, for example, a pot-belly or proportionally bigger hips and thighs.

If you have to make continual efforts to restrict the amount of food you eat or to exercise regularly to maintain a stable weight, the chances are that your *Slimming System* is not working as well as it should. These signs also indicate that the *Slimming System* is now in need of urgent attention.

The New Way We Need to Lose Weight

We must realize that to lose weight in our chemically contaminated environment, we have to adapt the way we diet to the new situation we find ourselves dealing with. Thus, today, dieting should always be undertaken with detoxification. In fact, dieting without detox is not just ineffective but potentially dangerous.[30]

The benefits of combining diet and detox include permanent weight loss as well as a whole raft of other health benefits, because by removing the toxic chemicals that make you fat, you will also do away with the ones that appear to make you ill.

So now we know how chemicals damage our natural *Slimming System*. The next step is to find out which are the worst offenders. As it is clearly no longer possible to remove all synthetic chemicals from our lives, we need to devise a plan to reduce our exposure to the most fattening of these chemicals and to find ways to increase their rate of removal from our bodies.

And I now have the pleasure of introducing Part Two, which will start you on your way to lasting slimness. By learning which chemicals are the most fattening, their uses, and where they tend to be found, you will be well on your way to discovering the real secret of how to lose weight in the twenty-first century.

Part Two

CHEMICAL CALORIES

6

All About *Chemical Calories*:
The Dieter's No. 1 Enemy

This chapter presents some of the most innovative material in the book. For the first time ever, the doors have been thrown wide open to a completely new way for us to identify the most fattening chemicals in the food chain and the environment, singling them out from the hundreds of thousands of others that are less fattening so that we can avoid them. And while total exclusion is out of the question, the good news is that we can all be far more selective.

Cutting out the most fattening chemicals first will enable us to make an enormous difference with comparatively little effort. And as we begin to see the weight loss benefits for ourselves, we can take a more informed view about limiting the chemicals in our food as well as considering how far to go in removing potentially fattening products from our homes. In the long term, we can also make educated decisions about how to choose less fattening products or materials when the time comes to replace existing items. So how can all this be achieved?

Well, there is a key, and the key is the *Chemical Calorie*.

The Origins of the *Chemical Calorie*

The idea of the *Chemical Calorie* was first conceived a few months after my initial discovery that chemicals could make us fatter. By then I had already come across a very large number of chemicals that produced fattening effects, but it was becoming clearer by the day that the ability of these different chemicals to fatten varied greatly.

As there were so many different kinds of these substances, it became more and more evident that I had to find some way to rank them according to their "fattening" ability. This kind of ranking system would enable people to tackle the problem head on, since by knowing which were the worst offenders, they could avoid the foods or places in which they were found.

It was while I was turning all this over in my mind that I decided to take my young sons to their favorite play area. As they were romping around, I found myself toying with several different words on a piece of scrap paper. Initially, I got nowhere and stopped to take a break, bought myself and my boys a drink, then after a while returned to take a second look at what I had been doing. Then it happened.

The words *chemical* and *calorie* placed accidentally side by side suddenly leapt out at me. Eureka! I had inadvertently written down the name of a totally new unit, one that would provide a revolutionary way of measuring the fattening ability of the chemicals in virtually every conceivable kind of food and household product.

At that moment, the *Chemical Calorie* was born.

Chemical Calories Versus Traditional Calories

Chemical Calories are very different from calories in the traditional sense. Conventional calories are simply units of energy. Based on your body's ability to convert food into energy, food can be described as having a certain caloric value. So the more conventional calories in a food, the more energy the food will produce, which is why fats possess more calories than carbohydrates, because the body can extract more energy from fats. So how do *Chemical Calories* work, in comparison?

Chemical Calories produce their fattening effect in an entirely different way. Unlike foods, these toxic chemicals have no inherent energy value. They contain no conventional calories as such. So how can they make us fat?

What they do have is an ability to slow down and disrupt the efficiency of our *Slimming System*. If our *Slimming System* is less able to work, our body will become less able to convert foods into energy. So the "leftover" foods, which the body is now unable to convert into useful energy, end up being stored as fat.

Effectively, then, the fattening ability of a chemical can be measured by the degree of damage caused to the *Slimming System,* and it is this damage that is measured in units of *Chemical Calories*. As a result, the chemicals that produce more damage to the *Slimming System* will generally contain more *Chemical Calories* than those that bring about less damage.

Finding *Chemical Calorie* Values for Different Foods

Just as a quarter cup of butter has more conventional calories than a quarter cup of rice, a fixed amount of one chemical could make you much fatter than the same amount of another chemical, if it possesses more *Chemical Calories*. As a result, foods that contain large amounts of the chemicals that I have assessed to be particularly fattening will be rated very high in *Chemical Calories*; if you want to lose weight, these are the foods to avoid. Foods that contain lower amounts of less damaging chemicals will have a medium or low *Chemical Calorie* rating.

You will see from the *Chemical Calorie* food charts in Chapter 15 how the rating system works. These totally revolutionary food charts show which foods are more likely to contain the chemicals that make us fatter. Now I will tell you how this major step forward was actually achieved.

Identifying the Most Fattening Chemicals

There are currently hundreds of thousands of different chemicals in use. As it would be virtually impossible to analyze them all separately, the first thing I did was divide them into groups that shared similar features—for example, all the different types of organophosphate pesticides were analyzed together.

Once I had established the main chemical groups involved, I turned my attention to identifying the most important parts of the *Slimming System*. I found that these included the major hormones involved in weight control; fat, protein, carbohydrate, and energy metabolism; and the ability to exercise.[1]

Using information gleaned from thousands of scientific papers, I then scored each group of chemicals according to the extent to which they appeared to cause damage to each individual part of our *Slimming System*.

Last, the overall total figure was multiplied by a figure relating to the time taken for the chemical to be excreted from our bodies. The final figure obtained from these calculations was the actual *Chemical Calorie* rating.

Despite being estimates, my *Chemical Calorie* ratings appeared to correlate remarkably well with each chemical's ability to fatten. Virtually all the chemicals with low *Chemical Calorie* ratings tended not to be strongly associated with weight gain, whereas those with high or very high ratings appeared to actively cause weight gain. The higher the *Chemical Calorie* rating, the stronger the fattening effect seemed to be.

Of course it would have been better to try to measure this effect in the laboratory, but to obtain such information would have involved many years of research and great cost. Even then, we would still be left with the potential problem of working out how all these chemicals react with one another to possibly magnify their fattening effects. Until someone can directly measure these effects, these estimated ratings provide a unique way for us to determine where the most fattening chemicals can be found in our food and environment right now, instead of in ten or twenty years.

At this point, it's time to introduce the groups of chemicals that appear to be causing the most trouble with our weight.

The *Chemical Calorie* "Hit List"

Based on the above estimates, I have found the most fattening groups of chemicals to be as follows:

First place	Organochlorine pesticides (DDT, lindane, etc.)
Second place	Organochlorine (PCBs) and organobromine (PBBs and PBDEs) industrial pollutants
Third place	Heavy metals (e.g., cadmium)
Fourth place (joint)	Other pesticides (organophosphates, carbamates, etc.)
Fourth place (joint)	Synthetic materials (plasticizers, PVC, styrenes)
Fifth place	Solvents (e.g., trichloroethylene [TCE])

You may recognize some of the names of these chemicals, not only because I may have previously mentioned them but also because they include substances that are very widely used. As time goes on, I will be cross-checking these results, so the actual rankings may change somewhat as I do further research, but I've done more than enough research already to know that these groups of chemicals will remain among the worst offenders.

The good news is that by having this ranking, not only do we now know which substances to avoid, but it now also becomes possible to create ways to specifically target their removal from our bodies. So let's find out more about these chemicals on our hit list.

Organohalogens (Organochlorines and Organobromines)

I have previously introduced the best-known examples of this group of chemicals, the organochlorines, in Chapter 3, but you can see that they need to be described further because of their top ranking and widespread presence.

In the earlier part of the twentieth century, organochlorines were used very extensively as pesticides. Though the use of some members of this group has largely been stopped in developed countries, they are still found virtually everywhere—in our bodies, in our food, and in the environment—because of their stability.

Just because some organochlorines have been banned, it doesn't mean that we are not still being exposed to them. Some countries still produce "banned" organochlorine pesticides in large quantities, shipping them overseas where they can easily be used on food crops. They may then be "returned" to us in imported foodstuffs. Our local foods are still being treated with other pesticides from this group, and all the time even more organochlorine pesticides are entering the food chain through environmental contamination. The relevant message is that despite their production being gradually reduced, they are still very much out there and will be for many future generations.

Since organochlorine pesticides appear to be the most powerfully fattening chemicals around us, I believe their avoidance and elimination from our bodies is essential for achieving permanent weight loss.

The second most fattening chemicals, known as *polychlorinated biphenyls*, or PCBs, are extremely common, not just in food but in water and in the air. Because of their extreme stability, PCBs used to be popular as electrical insulators. Since being banned (because of their extreme persistence), they have become some of the most common environmental pollutants and contaminate a whole range of foods.[2]

The *polybrominated biphenyls* (PBBs) and *polybrominated diphenyl ethers* (PBDEs) compounds are structurally very similar to PCBs and DDT, and thus extremely stable as well as potentially highly toxic.[3] They have been used to lower the flammability of an extensive range of products. In fact, it is illegal *not* to treat certain goods—upholstered furniture, for example—with flame retardants! Despite environmental concerns about their use, as yet they have not been banned.

Other Fattening Chemicals

As you can see from the hit list, there are many other types of chemicals that appear to possess a powerful fattening effect. Beginning with the heavy metals, cadmium in particular is high in *Chemical Calories.* Although the fattening effect of this group in general does not appear to be as marked as that of the organochlorines, it still ranks very high because of the chemicals' extreme persistence—once we have absorbed heavy metals, they tend to remain in our bodies for many years.[4]

Next comes a large number of pesticides commonly used on our foods, such as organophosphates and carbamates. The fact that many of these chemicals have also been used as growth promoters testifies to their weight-enhancing potential (see Chapter 3).

Certain kinds of synthetic materials also appear to contain a large amount of *Chemical Calories,* in particular the styrenes (as in polystyrene).[5]

Finally, there is a whole range of solvents, such as trichloroethylene (TCE), the dry-cleaning solvent, and those used widely in industry and in paints, glues, and cleaning fluids, which possess moderate amounts of *Chemical Calories.*[6]

I have found that the longer these chemicals remain in the body, the bigger the problem they tend to cause. So the chemicals that last for years, rather than days and weeks, will possess far more *Chemical Calories* than those less persistent substances. However, because we tend to be exposed to so many substances, such as solvents, even the shorter-lived ones can still cause a significant problem. If you want to know more about these substances, their uses, and where they are found, see Appendix A.

Determining the *Chemical Calorie* Content of Foods

One of my main goals in working out the *Chemical Calorie* ratings of chemicals was to discover which foods make us fat by virtue of their chemical content. I admit that a mixture of personal and public interest was there right from the beginning; after all, who wants to eat foods that could be making her or him fatter? In order to work out the *Chemical Calorie* content of a food, we need to know two things: first, the *Chemical Calorie* rating for all the individual chemicals detected in the food; second, the levels at which these chemicals are present. As national food agencies conduct regular tests to measure the levels of pesticide residues on commonly consumed foods,[7] it should be relatively easy to use these data to work out the overall *Chemical Calorie* content of a food or drink—and this is exactly what I have done.

The *Chemical Calorie* value of a food can then be reached by multiplying the *Chemical Calorie* rating for each particular chemical by the amount of that chemical detected in the food tested. If there are multiple chemicals present, then the *Chemical Calorie* value of the food is the sum of these values. And there you have it!

Chemical Calorie Charts

I can tell you that when I first worked out the *Chemical Calorie* content of a whole range of foods, no one was more interested in the outcome of these calculations than I. And when I saw the results, I began to see some of our everyday foods in a completely new light. It was quite frankly shocking: Many of the foods that we have been told for years are extremely healthy revealed themselves to be anything but!

The aim of these charts is not to stop people from eating these foods completely but to reduce their exposure to the most contaminated versions of them or to find ways of preparing them in order to make them less fattening.

The charts in Chapter 15 will, I hope, help you reach that goal. They reveal which foods are very low, low, medium, high, and very high in *Chemical Calories,* and the data are presented in a manner similar to that of ordinary calorie charts. Better still, most of the foods that you would typically find in ordinary calorie charts are also listed, including a wide range of meat and meat products, dairy products, fish, fruit, vegetables, grain products, oils and fats, and certain processed foods.

This information should be particularly welcome, as food labels are not yet required by law to give any information about pesticides and other such chemicals used during production and packaging. At present, it is simply impossible to assess how contaminated your food will be just from reading the wrapper.

Hopefully, my user-friendly *Chemical Calorie* charts will help change all that. They will let you see at a glance how foods vary in their *Chemical Calorie* levels. Use this as a guide to help you discover which foods are likely to be the most contaminated, which tend to be the safest, and when it is necessary to buy organic (foods produced with a minimum of artificial chemicals).

Although most organic foods are low in *Chemical Calories,* you will still need to watch out for the few that can be relatively contaminated from environmental pollutants, such as certain fish and animal products.

The good news is that you can now lose weight just by choosing the less contaminated food option. No deprivation is required. Painless dieting, after all these years of suffering from hunger and repetitive meals—what could be better than that?

Chemical Calories in Nonfood Products

When we eat food, we absorb most of the *Chemical Calories* it contains so effectively that we know exactly how many *Chemical Calories* we are being exposed to. But when we absorb *Chemical Calories* from the environment, we breathe them into our lungs and absorb them through our skin. Because these modes of absorption are more difficult to measure, it is more difficult to estimate precisely the amounts of *Chemical Calories* we take in from nonfood products.

However, it is possible to get an idea of the level of *Chemical Calories* in specific materials such as paint, carpet, or cosmetics by looking at what the product is made of. This, in combination with the way the product is used, enables us to determine which nonfood products are more likely than others to expose us to higher levels of *Chemical Calories*.

Whether you follow some or all the recommendations I have given you, all the advice that follows will be of immense value, since it provides a relatively easy way to help you lose weight that doesn't involve any food deprivation or discomfort. Not only will cutting down on *Chemical Calories* help you lose weight and stay slim for life, but it will also help lift the toxic burden off your body and boost your health for years to come. Now that's certainly worth striving for!

What Makes Strawberries More "Fattening" Than Avocados? Which Foods Are Highest in *Chemical Calories?*

It used to be so much easier to work out which foods were fattening and which were not. We were told that if we counted the conventional calorie content of foods and did not exceed recommended figures, we could control our weight. In fact, that's what we're still told.

We see calorie counts on chocolate bars and yogurt cartons. We see calorie counts at the top of recipes. We see calorie counts in endless numbers of magazines. We are bombarded with the words *low-calorie* and *low-fat* on "diet" food packaging and advertising. Calories are everywhere! They are so ingrained in Western culture that it is understandably difficult for somebody brought up in this environment to accept that there might be another way of thinking, much less to actually believe it. But look at the facts presented here and come to your own conclusions. And then try it out.

You will find the information in this chapter totally liberating. It will allow you for the first time to make more informed decisions about how to choose foods low in *Chemical Calories.* After telling you how foods come to be so contaminated, I then reveal the top twelve most contaminated foodstuffs—the "dirty dozen" on the scale of most fattening foods. Following this, I review all the major food groups, identifying some foods as higher in

Chemical Calories than others, exposing the worst offenders and explaining what makes them apparently so bad.

Armed with this information, with the advice on how to lower your intake of *Chemical Calories* given in the next two chapters, and finally with the full *Chemical Calorie* charts in Chapter 15, you will be completely capable of dramatically reducing your exposure to *Chemical Calories* from food.

While I accept that all this might take a bit of getting used to, the good news is that for the first time ever you now have the know-how that will help you on your way to achieving safe and permanent weight loss. Now that's something really positive.

So How Can Strawberries Be More Fattening Than Avocados?

Take a look at any calorie chart, and you will discover that strawberries are extremely low in conventional calories while avocados are very high. Even to suggest that the reverse is true seems to go against absolutely everything that we have been taught.

So what makes strawberries more fattening than avocados? The answer is very simple. Strawberries have far more *Chemical Calories* than avocados do. This is because strawberries are a relatively fragile food crop that tends to be sprayed repeatedly with "fattening" pesticides and preservatives to maximize its survival in the field and on the shelf. On the other hand, the avocado is a much more robust crop that needs hardly any active intervention at all. As a result, it is much lower in *Chemical Calories*. So from the *Chemical Calorie* viewpoint, strawberries are more fattening than avocados.

Food Is the Major Source of Chemical Contamination

For the majority of you, who do not come into contact with large amounts of chemicals at work, food will be your main source of chemical exposure, since most *Chemical Calories* creep into your body unseen on the food that you eat. And once they are inside your gut, your body is forced to deal with them, either by storing them or by breaking them down, if indeed it can.

You have already seen that the weight of people who make the "mistake" of eating modest amounts of even one kind of highly contaminated food can be affected. If you go back to some of the studies quoted in Chapter 3, you will see that they show that just by eating average amounts of contaminated fish, ordinary people can actually become fatter. If just one food can be found to have such a significant effect, you can imagine the effect that all the other polluted foods could be having on our weight.

To lose weight, we need to know which foods out of the multitude available are the most fattening, so that we can cut them out of our diet, replacing them with safer and less fattening foods.

Where the Chemicals in Our Foods Come From

How do chemicals actually get into the food that we eat? It would be relatively easy if all the chemicals in our food were from deliberately added chemicals, such as pesticides or preservatives. However, life is never that simple. In real life, chemicals can enter our food in a variety of different ways:

- Pesticides, additives, preservatives, or colorants are deliberately sprayed onto or added to food crops.
- Farm animals are treated with drugs or hormones and have antibiotics added to their feed.
- Food crops or animals are affected by environmental pollution.
- Chemicals leach out into foods from packaging materials.

Despite the variety of ways in which chemicals enter foods, government agencies tend mainly to test and monitor the levels of food contamination caused by pesticides. Because of the availability of this information, in combination with the extensive testing in this area, I have based all the following figures on this pesticide information alone.

While this information will give you an excellent guideline for judging the potential level of *Chemical Calories* from pesticides in a product, it will not be able to give you the total figure. However, to help you make a more accurate assessment, I will also provide you with loads of relevant advice that will help you limit your exposure from all forms of food-borne *Chemical Calories*. Don't worry; once you know what to look for, it will become quite easy to spot the potential problem areas.

The Dirty Dozen

Now we have arrived at the nitty gritty: Which of all our foods are the most contaminated with *Chemical Calories*? I have created the list below from the four most recent consecutive individual reports available from the U.S. Food and Drug Administration (FDA) Total Diet Study.[1] This is an ongoing food-testing program that regularly monitors pesticide residues in food. The Total Diet Study is designed to estimate the average amount of pesticides consumed by people of all ages in their food. FDA personnel purchase foods from supermarkets or smaller grocery stores four times per year from each of four geographical regions of the country. The foods are prepared table ready, then analyzed for pesticide residues. In order to work out the *Chemical Calorie* lists, I used a year's worth of data (four data sets from 1998 to 1999) taken from the Total Diet Study, as this was the most up-to-date information available to me.

At the No. 1 spot, as you can see, butter is according to my calculations the most contaminated food *Chemical Calorie*–wise, with the others following in descending order.

1. Butter, regular salted
2. Salmon, steaks or fillets, fresh or frozen, baked
3. Spinach, fresh or frozen, boiled
4. Strawberries, raw
5. Cream cheese
6. Raisins
7. Apple, red, raw, unpeeled
8. Dill cucumber pickles
9. Summer squash, fresh or frozen, boiled

10. Green peppers
11. Collards, fresh or frozen, boiled
12. Processed cheese, U.S.

Rather than explain each result individually, it will be easier to go through all the major food groups, starting with those containing foods with the highest levels of *Chemical Calories*. For each group I'll explain how the foods come to be contaminated and suggest particular foods in each group that are also likely to be particularly high or low in *Chemical Calories*.

DAIRY AND EGG PRODUCTS

Butter is in the unenviable position at the top of the list of dirty-dozen foods. But it is not just butter, as two other dairy products also appear in the dirty dozen. This in itself should serve as a severe warning about including a lot of fat-rich dairy products in your diet.

The reason they rank at the top is because of their levels of organochlorines. Dairy foods tend to be vulnerable to this particular kind of contamination since one of the few ways in which animals can rid themselves of persistent chemicals is by expelling them in their milk or in their offspring. Chickens and other farmed birds can also off-load persistent chemicals or, indeed, any other chemical they are exposed to in their eggs.

As most of the *Chemical Calories* tend to be stored in fats,[2] the highest levels will reside in fat-rich foods such as butter, cream cheese, and other cheeses. Consequently, dairy products that are lower in fats tend to be lower in *Chemical Calories*, for example, skim or partially skim milk, low-fat yogurt or cottage cheese.

FISH AND SHELLFISH

Now prepare yourself, as the following may come as a shock to many of you. At second place in the dirty dozen comes salmon. Yes, I am afraid it's true that salmon, which is generally regarded as a healthy food and full of nutritionally enhancing oils, appears to be extremely high in *Chemical Calories*. So how has this crazy state of affairs come to pass in which fish—one of our most nutritious and beloved foods, particularly by dieters—has been defiled?

The heart of this problem is the large-scale contamination of our lakes and oceans with chemicals such as organochlorines—in particular, DDT and dioxins. These toxic and extremely persistent chemicals have invaded every environment on the face of the earth by virtue of their ability to evaporate into the air, circulate in the atmosphere, and be carried back down to the ground in rain, resulting in the pollution of most water sources. Despite this, some oceans tend to be more polluted than others, and consequently the fish from them will be more contaminated.

Since these chemicals are extremely fat soluble, they are easily absorbed across the surface of fish gills and thereby enter the fish. They will also cling to particles in the water such as plankton, which are then eaten in vast quantities by fish.[3] Those fish may well carry the chemical in their bodies for good.

Carnivorous predators like salmon and trout are helpless "victims" of this pollution because they eat large quantities of small fish, thus further ratcheting up the levels of contamination (a process called *biomagnification*), since none of the species involved is capable of breaking down and eliminating these persistent chemicals.

But if you are a fish lover, don't become too despondent. There is some good news, as noncarnivorous fish, which includes many kinds of fish with white flesh such as cod, tend to be much less polluted. This is because these fish feed lower in the food chain. In addition, they also have a much lower fat content and so have less of a buildup of fat-loving pollutants. And based on the FDA data used, shellfish also appear to be less contaminated by pesticides and so appear in my charts to be relatively low in *Chemical Calories*. But due to the fact that shellfish can often contain relatively high levels of heavy metals and other chemical contaminants, they may in the future be found to contain higher levels of *Chemical Calories* than these pesticide charts initially suggest.

VEGETABLES AND VEGETABLE PRODUCTS

Rather than being derived from environmental contamination, as in the previous groups, the main source of *Chemical Calories* in vegetables tends to be pesticides that are deliberately added during the growing process or used to prolong life in storage. The factors controlling how often a vegetable crop is sprayed with chemicals, and ultimately how high the chemical levels will be, depend on the fragility of the crop during growth and storage, whether it is a cash crop, and how important it is for the vegetable to look good. The more fragile a crop tends to be, the more likely it is that chemicals will be used multiple times to prevent damage and to stop the crop from going moldy in storage.

Unfortunately, one of the most heavily used pesticides for vegetables worldwide also happens to have been previously used as a growth promoter (organophosphates),[4] so it is not too surprising that a large number of vegetables are significantly high in *Chemical Calories*. If it is important for a vegetable to be free from blemishes, then chances are it will be treated more intensely.

After being applied, many of the chemicals can remain on the surface of the foods. This is confirmed by the fact that baked potatoes prepared in their jackets tend to be high in *Chemical Calories,* but peeled potatoes tend to be much lower. So although vegetables appear to rank relatively high, the simple act of peeling them can dramatically lower the level of foodborne *Chemical Calories.*

Similarly, removing the outside leaves on a head of lettuce dramatically lowers the overall level of *Chemical Calories.* However, if the vegetable consists of leaves that aren't bound together tightly, such as collard greens or spinach, you can't lower the *Chemical Calorie* content as dramatically just by removing the outside leaves, as most of the leaves will have been directly exposed to pesticides.

Salad vegetables, such as cucumber, carrots, and radishes, which tend to be consumed raw, appeared to contain very significant amounts of *Chemical Calories.* This would make these apparently healthy low-calorie "diet" foods potentially fattening *Chemical Calories*–wise unless you are careful to remove the peel.

Finally, the summer squashes that rank ninth may have gotten there despite being peeled, as certain chemicals don't just stay on the outside of the vegetable but are able to penetrate it. Consequently, no amount of preparation would be truly effective in lowering their *Chemical Calorie* rating.

FRUIT AND FRUIT PRODUCTS

Back again to the succulent strawberry, it really does seem a shame that such an innocent food should be so relatively contaminated with *Chemical Calories*. As with vegetables, the main source of contamination of fruit appears to be the deliberate spraying of pesticides at different stages of the growing process. In other words, these are chemicals that are deliberately added during the growing process or to prolong life in storage.

I suppose you can understand to some extent why these relatively "fragile" crops appear to be sprayed more intensively, as fruit tends to look more appealing and therefore fetches a better price when it has an unblemished exterior. And farming, after all, is a business.

So let's get down to the nitty-gritty of which fruits have the highest levels of *Chemical Calories*. Of all the fruits, the poor old strawberry ranks fourth in the dirty dozen, which is a terrible blow for all fruit lovers and to me personally, as it is one of my all-time favorite fruits. The next two fruits that make it into the top twelve are raisins and red apples (raw), which rank sixth and seventh, respectively. These are closely followed by soft fruits such as peaches, sweet cherries, and plums. Again, the problem here is that these fruits tend not to be peeled before being tested. And as the majority of chemicals reside mainly on the outside, these fruits will tend to be much higher in *Chemical Calories* than fruits that have to be peeled before eating, such as oranges and bananas.

Just to highlight the value of peeling fruit in cutting the levels of *Chemical Calories*, there is another interesting comparison between the U.K. *Chemical Calorie* charts and the U.S. charts. In the United Kingdom, where the whole fruit, peel and all, is tested, certain fruits, such as oranges, rank very high there mainly because of the presence of pesticides on the orange peels. But here in the United States, oranges are relatively low in *Chemical Calories* because the fruit is prepared for eating before it is tested—that is, the peel is removed. As people tend not to eat the peel unless they are eating marmalade, and as most of the chemicals detected tend to stay on the peel, the inner part tends to be far less contaminated.[5]

So it seems that peeling fruit before eating can be an extremely simple way to considerably lower the overall level of *Chemical Calories*.

CONDIMENTS

Although you might wonder why this category has been included, as the amounts of these foods that are consumed tend to be relatively small, I believe this mixed group of food merits inclusion because many of us regularly use lots of sauces and pickles to make our foods more exciting. Consequently, for some people this group will constitute a significant proportion of their diet.

The main "problem" food in this group was the dill cucumber pickle, which came in at eighth place. Sweet cucumber pickles also appeared to contain significant amounts of *Chemical Calories*. On the plus side, the ubiquitous tomato ketchup appeared to be relatively low in *Chemical Calories*.

CONVENIENCE FOODS

This group is very much a mixed bag of foods, ranging from pizza to coleslaw. The problem comes in estimating the *Chemical Calorie* values of these foods, due to the variety of food combinations available. For instance, one brand of lasagne could contain a much larger amount of meat sauce than another brand that contains more white sauce. Because of this huge variability, it is very hard to generalize about what makes some convenience foods higher in *Chemical Calories* than others.

When I buy convenience foods, I determine which kind of food forms the bulk of the meal, and if that food is potentially high in *Chemical Calories*, then I treat the whole meal as if it were in that category. The same rule of thumb holds true for eating out: If you take into account all the main constituents of the meal, you will have an idea how high a level of *Chemical Calories* it contains.

NUTS AND BEANS

Most surprising was the number of different chemicals found in peanut butter. Not only were pesticides present, but so too were quite a few solvents. In fact, peanut butter almost made the dirty dozen but was just beaten by the American processed cheese that sneaked in at twelfth place.

Fortunately, the pinto and kidney beans tested performed much better, registering low amounts of *Chemical Calories*. This is excellent news, as beans are naturally rich in "slimming" nutrients such as vitamins, minerals, and proteins. Another benefit is that they are also packed full of that great detoxer—soluble fiber.

MEATS AND POULTRY

Meats vary far more in their *Chemical Calorie* content than do most other foods. This is because animals are exposed to a larger number of potential sources of contamination. Animals are affected not only by the environment they grew up in, but also by the food they have been fed or by the substances they have been treated with in their lifetime. These differences can lead to a huge variation in the amount of *Chemical Calories* in meat products. For instance, meat produced by one farmer may be relatively high in *Chemical Calories*, whereas the same kind of meat from livestock raised in a different place or fed fewer chemicals may be low in *Chemical Calories*.

The amount of fat in meat also appears to have some relationship to the overall *Chemical Calorie* loading. This is because most animals tend to store chemicals that they cannot metabolize in their body fat. Meats low in fat tend to be lower in *Chemical Calories* from pesticides—chicken and turkey being good examples.

On the subject of poultry, something you must bear in mind is that some animals, particularly those farmed intensively, are very likely to have been treated with antibacterial growth promoters. As half the antibacterial agents administered in the United States are used to enhance growth in animals, their influence on the levels of *Chemical Calories* in the meat of chickens, their eggs, and meat from any animal raised intensively needs to be considered when eating meats and poultry. To keep the chances of contamination down, I would recommend buying either organically produced meats or meats produced using less intensive farming methods. I do this myself, as I buy beef from a local farmer. Although it is not certified organic,

I know that the animals are raised without chemicals and that the major portion of their diet is comprised of fresh hill grass!

FATS, OILS, AND SHORTENINGS

This is an interesting category, as it consists of oils derived both from animals and from vegetables. From looking at the previous groups, you can see that the ways *Chemical Calories* get into animals vary slightly from the ways they get into plants.

In plant-based oils, the major source of contamination is deliberately added pesticides, such as those sprayed on vegetable-oil crops. But for the animal fats and shortenings, the most important sources of *Chemical Calories* are environmental exposure and the extent to which the animals' food supplies are contaminated. As these levels can vary greatly, the overall amount of *Chemical Calories* in fats, particularly animal fats, is relatively difficult to predict and makes using them potentially riskier.

GRAIN PRODUCTS

The average U.S. citizen consumes a large proportion of bread and cereal in his or her diet each year, so any contamination of grain products will have a sizable impact because of quantity alone. Fortunately, though, because grain tends to be more processed, the levels of *Chemical Calories* found in grain-based products tend to be comparatively low.

Grain is routinely sprayed with chemicals that speed up or slow down the growth of crops. During the growth cycle, it is extensively sprayed with potentially fattening insecticides, then after it has been harvested and put in storage, it could be exposed to even more pesticides to prevent infestations. It is also relatively common for organophosphates, in the form of a fine powder, to be mixed into piles of grain and then just not removed at a later date.

Bizarrely, products made with whole-meal flour—which we tend to think of as being more healthy—tend to have larger residues than processed white flour, with the highest levels of *Chemical Calories* being found in bran. This is because the residues cling to the outside of the grains. So, as a general rule, the more processed the grains are, the lower they are in *Chemical Calories*—and the lower they will be in nutritional value.

BEVERAGES

Now this will come as a relief for all you coffee and tea drinkers out there. Out of all the groups of foods tested, as a whole, beverages came out on top, or rather they were found to be the least contaminated by *Chemical Calories*. And despite wine being the highest in this group, compared to all the other beverages, the levels found in wine were comparatively very low. Fortunately for wine lovers, grapes grown for wine are mashed and thus do not need to be treated with the chemicals designed to preserve their succulent "good looks." So cheers to all of you!

Traditional Dieting Can Be Bad for You!

Chemical Calorie ratings clearly show that many of the foods traditionally associated with dieting—salad vegetables, fruit, and fish—are likely to be very heavily contaminated by chemicals. So by eating a much larger proportion of these foods in your diet, you would in all probability be exposing yourself to higher levels of *Chemical Calories* than you would when not actively dieting, defeating the whole purpose of trying to lose weight!

An even more sinister possibility emerges as well. The so-called safe doses of pesticides in a typical American diet could easily be exceeded by dieters because of their tendency to eat more of these relatively heavily contaminated foods. In that case, not only will dieters be more likely to become fatter in the long term, but their risks of developing chemically related diseases could also increase. This may even explain why people whose weight fluctuates frequently are at a much higher risk of getting a broad range of different illnesses.

By now you will have realized that many of the foods you have previously eaten, in addition to any previous dieting attempts, may actually be the source of your continual struggle with your weight. But don't despair; it really is possible to repair the damage from the past as well as reduce your risk of future weight gain.

In the next chapter, I will tell you how to reduce your exposure to *Chemical Calories* while still eating the foods that you love. What better way could there be to lose weight for good?

8

Don't Panic, Go Organic: Getting the Most Benefit from Organic Foods

At this point you are probably reeling from the news that many of the foods you have been eating in order to lose weight in the past could have been having quite the opposite effect. You just have to be philosophical about this and accept that what is past is past, but at least you now appreciate this fact and can start doing something constructive about it.

Your goal should now be to eat the foods that contain the lowest possible levels of *Chemical Calories* without overdosing on conventional calories that can also pack on the weight. The two-pronged solution lies in eating a nutritionally balanced diet that is more organic. This chapter will explain what it means to be organic and how to recognize organic foods. It will also tell you why organic foods are generally much lower in *Chemical Calories* than "conventionally" grown foods and why they really do taste far better or, in other words, why in my opinion they rank among the best slimming foods you can eat!

So What Are Organic Foods?

Organic foods are simply foods that are grown without most of the synthetic chemicals used in conventional farming, with a minimum level, if any, of synthetic pesticides, antibiotics, growth hormone, or fertilizers—pretty much like the food humans were eating since time began up to the beginning of this century.

As organic fruits and vegetables are grown with more stringent rules governing the use of synthetic chemicals, they end up being much lower in *Chemical Calories* than their intensively grown counterparts. An in-depth study conducted by the Consumers' Union (CU)[1] has shown that this is true. One of the paper's coauthors, Edward Groth, Senior Scientist at CU, said, "We have shown that consumers who buy organic fruits and vegetables are exposed to just one-third as many residues as they'd eat in conventionally grown foods, and the residues are usually lower as well." He also found that food grown organically had fewer and generally lower levels of pesticide residues than food produced by conventional methods.

But hang on, you might say. If few chemicals are deliberately added, why should organic foods possess any *Chemical Calories* at all? Well, unfortunately, due to the extensive presence of pollutants in our environment, neither conventionally grown nor organically grown foods will ever be totally *Chemical Calorie*–free.

But how can you tell which foods are organic just by looking at them? To help you identify them, all organic produce available in stores should bear a special seal from the U.S. Department of Agriculture (USDA) certifying that it is organic. This is part of a brand-new strategy introduced in October 2002 to unify organic food production.

These new organic standards offer a national definition for the term *organic*. They detail the methods, practices, and substances that can be used in producing and handling organic crops and livestock as well as processed foods. You can access this information at the following website address: www.ams.usda.gov/nop/. The new USDA seals can be found on all food packaging that contains either 100 percent organic or 96 percent organic ingredients. All producers of organic foods must be accredited with the USDA to be able to use the seal.

Why Is Organic Food Different?

Probably the most important features distinguishing organic foods from conventionally grown foods are:

- Improved flavor and food texture.
- Increased nutritional content.
- Lower levels of toxic heavy metals, organochlorines, and pesticides.

It wasn't until I tasted my first organically grown apple that I knew something was seriously wrong with our food industry. It was so different from all the other apples I had eaten in the previous twenty years. They had left a strange aftertaste in my mouth, but the organic apple tasted simply great, taking me back to my childhood, when we picked our own apples from the trees in my parents' garden. From then on, I was hooked.

Since then, my understanding also has totally changed. Instead of marveling over the superficial beauty of conventional foods, I think about how many chemicals the farmer used to get them to look good and grow large. I am now even happy when I find the occasional bug on organic fruits and vegetables, because it is evidence that my food has not been sprayed with nasties. If that bug can survive, then nothing on the food is likely to harm me.

Better Flavor and Superior Texture

You don't have to be a vegetarian or on a weight reduction program to enjoy organic produce. Foodies have already discovered that the taste and quality of organic foods are far superior. Fruit and vegetables taste sweeter, oats taste creamier, chocolate is sensational, and meat and chicken have real depth of flavor. Even pasta, rice, and bread taste slightly sweeter and more flavorful.

This is not just a marketing ploy. There are two very good reasons organic food really does taste better. First, organic produce tends to be higher in natural sugars (approximately 21 percent more than in conventionally grown foods).[2] This is thought to be because the chemicals and nitrates in fertilizers interfere with a plant's own metabolism, particularly by reducing its level of natural sugars. Without interference from excessive amounts of artificial fertilizers, organic foods with their higher levels of natural sugars really do taste sweeter.

Second, pesticides appear to alter the sensations the brain gets from the taste buds, distorting flavors when we eat, and also to damage our sense of smell. Common pesticides (such as carbamates) significantly reduce taste and smell, and can leave a metallic or bitter flavor in the mouth.[3]

The texture of organic meat also appears to be far superior. This is probably because the animals are raised slowly, are fed more natural foods, are not treated with growth hormone, and get more exercise. This appears to be most evident in pork and poultry, possibly due to the artificially forced growth rates in nonorganic meat production.

I've found the differences in meats to be most noticeable with organic bacon, which I think tastes out of this world. But don't just take my word for it, try it out for yourself!

Packed with Slimming Nutrients

It's official. According to a scientific study by nutritionist Anne-Marie Mayer, based on published data from *The Composition of Foods,* a comprehensive study of the content of all major foods dating back to 1940, conventionally grown fruits and vegetables have been found to have fewer nutrients than they had fifty years ago.[4] It seems that modern farming methods, using large amounts of agrochemicals and artificial fertilizers, have effectively depleted the soil of essential minerals. This means that the quantities of essential minerals in our foods have been reduced alarmingly. Levels of magnesium, iodine, potassium, zinc, calcium, and iron have plummeted, and as we desperately need these to power our natural *Slimming System,* this can directly influence our weight.

By comparison, a recent review of forty-one studies comparing organic and conventionally grown foods concluded that, overall, organic farming methods appear to produce foods that contain higher levels of minerals and vitamins.[5] This is thought to be because the soil is treated with naturally balanced fertilizers containing a more balanced spread of minerals. And in addition, organic crops tend to be more robust, because organically grown plant metabolism is less damaged by pesticides, so the plants can also produce more vitamins. In particular, vitamin C, which is a carbohydrate and so particularly at risk of damage in conventionally grown plants, tends to be found in higher quantities in organic foods.

But the differences don't stop there: The proteins found in organic fruits and vegetables are also of higher quality.[6] So by eating organically, your body can luxuriate in larger amounts of high-quality "slimming" nutrients that are vital in keeping your weight down and stable.

Fewer *Chemical Calories*

Our planet is so polluted now that it is not possible to reduce our intake of *Chemical Calories* to zero. All our crops are exposed to and contaminated by chemicals in the atmosphere and in particular by PCBs from air and rainwater. Organically grown foods are just as likely as nonorganic foods to be contaminated in this way.

However, organically grown fruits and vegetables are far less polluted by *Chemical Calories* added during growth and storage. In addition, natural farming methods mean that organically grown crops tend to be less polluted by heavy metals and artificial fertilizers drawn from the soil.[7] Contaminated soil grows contaminated crops. So by buying organic fruits and vegetables, you will be reducing your *Chemical Calorie* exposure to the lowest levels possible.

Buying organically raised animals and organic dairy products will also help to seriously reduce the *Chemical Calories* in your diet. Since additives in what an animal eats will build up in its body over time, meats and dairy products from animals that eat less contaminated food have fewer *Chemical Calories*. In addition, organically raised animals are not treated with growth-enhancing substances, so when you're eating a piece of organic steak or chicken, you know that it doesn't have unwanted residues of those same chemicals that could potentially affect your weight too.

Sadly, all animals raised for food can be particularly affected by environmental pollution. Certain environments are now so contaminated that the livestock kept there will have far higher levels of *Chemical Calories* than livestock from other areas, even if raised organically.

Why Doesn't Everyone Eat Organic Food?

If it is so good, why doesn't everybody eat organic food? Well, as with everything in life, there are pros and cons. Price and availability have been major barriers for many people in the past, though this is changing. To help you get more of a feel for the issues, some of the most commonly quoted reasons for buying organic foods are:

- Generally much lower levels of *Chemical Calories* (to aid weight control).
- Higher levels of essential nutrients (to boost the *Slimming System,* your health, and possibly even your time on this planet).
- Environmentally friendly farming causes far less pollution.
- Organic farming appears to be more humane for animals.
- Organic food has superior taste.
- A lower toxic chemical intake will enhance rather than injure your general health.

Some disadvantages of organic food include:

- Generally 20 to 30 percent more expensive than conventionally produced food.
- Limited availability in shops and supermarkets.
- A smaller choice of foods (particularly convenience foods).
- Reduced shelf life.
- Sometimes less visually appealing.
- Few organic restaurants for eating out.
- Increased preparation time, since meals are mostly made from fresh ingredients.

It seems quite clear now that eating totally organically is the healthiest and most ideal way to lose weight, and practically everything I have suggested on my diet is now available organically. But can everyone eat organic all the time? Of course not. Now that organic products are more readily available, it is much easier than before, but it would be too difficult for many of us to be absolutely strict about it. But whatever you can do to slash *Chemical Calories* will be a huge step forward.

Even if your diet consists of food that is 100 percent organic, the following chapter will still prove to be essential reading, because it also covers the ways in which even the purest foods can become contaminated with *Chemical Calories* on the long journey from shop to plate. So read on to discover yet more indispensable secrets about how to achieve a diet low in *Chemical Calories*.

9

Eating Fewer *Chemical Calories*: How to Choose, Store, and Prepare Your Food to Minimize *Chemical Calories*

So you have just gone out and bought your first supply of organic food. Well, congratulations! You are at the starting point of your transformation into a new, slimmer you. But in order to maximize your weight loss, you need to know that there is actually a bit more to it than just eating organic foods. However careful you are about the foods you buy, there are plenty of ways in which *Chemical Calories* can still sneak into your foods before you eat them, transforming even the purest of organic foods into a seething mass of synthetic chemicals.

This chapter will tell you not only how to avoid these extra unwanted *Chemical Calories* that enter our food after being produced but also how to reduce the *Chemical Calorie* loading of both conventionally grown and organically raised foods.

How to Select Food Low in *Chemical Calories*

After reading the previous chapters, and armed with your *Chemical Calorie* charts (see Chapter 15), you will now be able to determine which foods are high in *Chemical Calories* and which are not when you go shopping. And if it is just too expensive to buy organic versions of everything on your shopping list, you will be able to choose conventional products that are likely to be the least contaminated and limit your organic shopping.

To be honest, this is probably the most sensible way to go. As long as you abide by the advice in this chapter and in the rest of the book, you will still be able to achieve the body you want even if you have very little or no access to organic foods at all. You just need to put a bit more effort into ensuring that your foods are as low in *Chemical Calories* as you can reasonably make them.

To start you off, I would like to provide some general rules to help you select foods with the lowest possible levels of *Chemical Calories*:

- When it comes to animal products, buy organic or less intensively farmed produce whenever you can.
- Keep animal fats low: Choose low-fat milk and other diary products, and leaner meats, even if the food is organic. (Low fat is especially important if the produce is not organic.) Make sure that the low-fat food and any processed food that you buy is also low in additives.
- Soft fruits and more delicate vegetables are likely to be more polluted than robust fruits and vegetables that store well.

Why It Is Better to Keep Your Intake of Animal Fats Low

Limiting your consumption of animal fats is generally a sensible policy, because most environmental pollutants accumulate in animals and tend to be stored in their fatty tissues. So by cutting down on animal fats, you will be automatically reducing the amount of *Chemical Calories* transferred to your body.

While it is relatively easy to choose meat with less visible fat, or low-fat dairy products, it becomes much more difficult to determine how much and which kinds of fat have been used in processed foods. On the whole, if given the choice, select products made with vegetable oils, as they are potentially less risky than those with animal fats.

One more point: Whether you buy organic produce or not, it's important to realize that most pesticides tend to be absorbed into your body far more readily if they are mixed with fats.[1] Because of this, you can limit to some extent the amount of pesticides you absorb from a food by lowering the overall fat content of the meal.

For example, if you buy a mixed nonorganically grown salad, make sure that you serve it with low-fat or no-fat dressing. If you really love canned salmon or tuna but want to keep down the *Chemical Calories,* buy it stored in water rather than oil.

How to Reduce *Chemical Calories* in Food Preparation

As previously mentioned, you don't have to go organic to eat fewer *Chemical Calories* (although it helps); with the right know-how, you can dramatically reduce the number of *Chemical Calories* by preparing and cooking food in certain ways. And while these techniques are particularly useful for conventional foods, they will also ensure that you get the most benefit from your organic produce too.

WASHING AND CLEANING

The most obvious way to rid your fruit and vegetables of pesticide residues is to wash them off. There has actually been quite a significant amount of scientific investigation into the effectiveness of removing chemicals by washing produce in plain water and by washing in water with detergents. On the whole, the results appear to depend largely on the kind of chemicals present.[2] Some pesticides are designed to stay on the surface, but others are specifically intended to infiltrate into the very heart of the food. As you can imagine, washing will only deal with chemicals found on the surface. But it has variable success even within that group, as some chemicals are water soluble and will wash off with plain water, while others are fat soluble and can only be removed by using detergents. Fortunately, rather than using dishwashing detergent, it is now possible to buy naturally derived products that claim to specifically remove many surface toxins from fruits and vegetables.

Despite proving more effective in some cases than others, washing your fruit and vegetables is a good first line of defense. However, for foods that absorb a certain amount of chemicals, such as strawberries, grapes, oranges, peaches, spinach, and tomatoes, washing is a good start, but a significant amount of chemicals may remain.

PEELING

Compared to washing, peeling fruit and vegetables can be a dramatic way to lower the *Chemical Calorie* content of food. Take, for example, an orange. If the peel is included (as orange zest, for example), it is one of the most polluted of all foods, but the simple act of peeling it will reduce the *Chemical Calorie* count considerably. This is because most of the chemicals in an orange are in its thick skin.[3]

The same applies to apples: Unpeeled, they can be very highly contaminated, yet once the skin is removed, the contamination is radically reduced.[4] Although a peeled apple cannot compare in flavor and goodness to an organic apple—which you should feel free to eat, peel and all—it is far safer and contains significantly fewer *Chemical Calories* than an unpeeled conventionally grown apple.

The same holds for vegetables such as tomatoes and, in particular, potatoes. So if you are eating nonorganic fruit and vegetables, you can still make a really big difference by getting the peeler out.

PREPARING MEATS AND FISH

I've already talked about the ways that *Chemical Calories* can accumulate in animal fat, so you can see that by cutting off all visible fat as you prepare meat, poultry, or fish, the *Chemical Calorie* content could potentially be greatly reduced.[5] In the case of fish, it is particularly beneficial to remove the skin before cooking if there tends to be a lot of fat just underneath it, which should help make all you fish fans out there a bit happier.

Reducing *Chemical Calories* Through Cooking

Since heat can break down certain chemicals and can also lower levels of others, food is usually lower in *Chemical Calories* after it has been cooked. Generally speaking, the higher the temperature and the longer the food is cooked, the more effective cooking will be in reducing the overall *Chemical Calorie* level.[6] For example, if you are making marmalade with nonorganic oranges, cooking it for a long time in an open pan on top of the stove is much more effective than the quicker lower-temperature method using a microwave oven.[7]

At the other extreme, some foods, such as vegetables, are cooked for only a short time. Despite the brief cooking time, however, many of the chemicals will still be washed off into the water. So if the potential level of *Chemical Calories* present in the vegetables is high, it may be best not to use the leftover water for making gravies or sauces.[8]

Some chemicals are more heat stable than others and are not destroyed by cooking. Indeed, in some cases cooking can actually make less toxic chemicals more toxic (which appears to be the case with one of the pesticides commonly found on tomatoes).[9] This is one more reason to always peel fruits and vegetables.

The more persistent chemicals, such as the organochlorines, can be virtually unaffected by cooking, which is not too surprising in view of their heat-resistant properties.[10] Indeed, some of the synthetic additives and veterinary drug residues found in meats (such as products to treat animals for worms) may not be destroyed either.[11]

In these cases, the main benefit of cooking is to remove some of the fat from meats and fish, as most of the aforementioned persistent chemicals tend to remain in these fats. Grilling and throwing away the fat is one option. Roasting is another, provided that the fat is not used in gravy. Another way is to cook meat or fish in vegetable oil and then throw all the oil and fat away.

I do think it is sad that things have come to this, since natural animal fats can really improve the flavor of many dishes, but if you don't know how

112

badly the fats are contaminated, eliminating them as much as possible is probably your best option. If, on the other hand, you are sure that the meats are relatively "clean," all this becomes less essential.

Apart from the extra preparation involved, there is another downside to all this peeling and cooking. Even though these techniques can be very effective in lowering the total levels of *Chemical Calories,* they will also tend to lower the nutritional value of the food, as vitamins are particularly heat sensitive. If you choose to use these methods, you must ensure that you are still getting enough nutrients by using supplements as recommended in Chapter 15.

10

Pure Water,
Your Weight-Loss Friend

To maximize the full slimming benefit of lowering our intake of *Chemical Calories* from food, we need to cut back on all the other ways in which our bodies are exposed to potentially harmful toxins.

After food, water is one of the main sources of *Chemical Calories*. And as we are exposed to water in so many different aspects of our lives, we can't afford to let it bypass our scrutiny. If we do, it will be to the detriment of our figures and, of course, of our general well-being.

This chapter will explain how our water has come to be so polluted and will outline what we can do to lower the levels of *Chemical Calories* in our own domestic water supply. Then it will explain how we can accelerate weight loss simply by drinking lots of *Chemical Calorie*–free water. Sound good? Now find out why!

How Clean Is Your Water Supply?

Since the creation and wide-scale use of synthetic chemicals, somewhat shockingly, more than 350 synthetic chemicals have been detected in tap water.[1] Not surprising, many of these substances have also revealed themselves to be very high in *Chemical Calories.*

The alarming contamination of our water supplies has largely occurred in the last 100 years, following years of industrial, agricultural, and environmental pollution. As a direct result, every day, as we eat, drink, wash, cook, clean, and go about our daily lives, we will now be exposed to and absorb whichever chemicals happen to be in our water supplies at the time.

The level of contamination varies a lot, depending on where you live, but a certain number of chemicals can be found universally, and they include the following groups:

- Pesticides
- Heavy metals
- Solvents
- Industrial pollutants
- Environmental pollutants
- Synthetic materials

In order to even start to tackle the problem, we need to understand how these toxins get into our water in the first place. This will give us a better idea how to improve the quality of our existing water supplies as well as reduce future contamination at its source.

1. *Seepage from the surface*

Whenever we use chemicals on the land, for any reason, it will usually lead to pollution of our underground water sources as well as our rivers and oceans. Chemicals used to clear weeds or improve crops or poison pests seep into the earth, where they then pollute the groundwater. In addition, wind and rain sweep the chemicals off the surface of the land into the rivers and the sea.

The most obvious example is the contamination caused by pesticides sprayed on fields by farmers in the process of growing crops. Not surprisingly, year after year these pesticides end up in our drinking water.

2. *Industrial waste*

This is another huge source of toxic chemical contamination. Waste from factories is commonly poured into rivers, or it can enter the water supply from the atmosphere or leak out from ill-managed toxic waste dumps. Once chemicals enter the water supply, they can cause damage for a surprisingly long time. A prime example of a persistent pollutant is the dry-cleaning substance and industrial solvent trichloroethylene, which is also very high in *Chemical Calories.*

Another persistent pollutant, especially in the United States, is a chemical called MTBE (methyl, tertiary-butyl ether). It was added to fuel in the late '70s in an attempt to make gasoline burn cleaner, but it had no real effect on curbing air pollution. Still, no one expected it to cause real harm. Several years ago, however, the sleepy village of Napoleon, Michigan, was the scene of a major unwanted discovery. In the course of drilling a new well for the church, it was found that the groundwater was so contaminated that it was unsafe to drink. It appeared that the underground storage tanks of three gas stations had been leaking and that the gasoline had seeped into the local aquifer, contaminating most of the wells in the vicinity.[2] After the alert was sounded, many other regions also found themselves facing the same problem. Quite apart from the pollution issues, MTBE appears to be very high in *Chemical Calories.*[3]

3. *Intentional adding of chemicals*
Not all the contamination in our water is accidental, since certain chemicals, such as chlorine and aluminum, are deliberately added to the supply. Aluminum is added in water-processing plants to "clear" the water. Although it is not particularly high in *Chemical Calories,* it does damage some aspects of our *Slimming System,* and it has also been linked to Alzheimer's disease.[4] Chlorine is another chemical that is deliberately added to water as a disinfectant. Although it is not particularly high in *Chemical Calories,* chlorine binds to other chemicals, forming trihalomethanes, which are thought to be carcinogenic. It also destroys proteins in the hair and skin, and makes water taste, in my opinion, disgusting.

4. *Environmental pollution*
As mentioned previously, certain chemicals, such as PCBs and other organochlorines, can evaporate into the air, particularly in warm countries. They may then be carried around the world's atmosphere and fall back onto

the ground in cooler countries, particularly via rainfall. In this way, even the most remote water sources have become polluted.

5. *Contamination from water pipes and storage containers*

Sometimes the storage and distribution system itself can add significant amounts of *Chemical Calories* to our water. Lead pipes (although these are being replaced) can add significantly to the *Chemical Calorie* loading of water, as can certain pipes made from synthetic materials, such as PVC (polyvinyl chloride).[5]

So exactly how do we absorb *Chemical Calories* from water, and how can we reduce our exposure to them?

How Do We Absorb
Chemical Calories from Water?

Most people will think that the main way we absorb *Chemical Calories* from water is by drinking it. I certainly did before researching this book, but it wasn't long before I discovered that this is not the whole story. There are two very important but less recognized routes by which *Chemical Calories* in water can enter our bodies: via our skin and our lungs. In fact, about half of the chlorine we absorb from water is thought to be through the lungs and skin,[6] and this contamination occurs every time we take a shower or bath in contaminated water.

As chlorine is not the only chemical present in our bathwater, chances are that many others are absorbed in this way too. This illustrates the importance of pure water for bathing as well as drinking in order to keep our total exposure to *Chemical Calories* as minimal as possible.

The next obvious question is: How do we achieve this?

Reducing the Level of
Chemical Calories in Water

Fortunately, we can do quite a lot to lower the *Chemical Calorie* content of water. Let's start by outlining a few of these protective measures:

- Before using the water, let cold taps run for a few minutes to flush out any lead that has leached into the water from the pipes.
- Use only the cold tap for drinking water and cooking, as there is a greater probability that the hot water contains lead, asbestos, and other pollutants from the hot water tank, if you have one.
- Use water filters to filter both your drinking water and your household supply.

Many people now invest in a home water-treatment system to ensure that all the water they use is as pure as possible. Many different methods are currently used to clean up water, but I will concentrate on the more commonly used ones.

PITCHER FILTER

The most commonly used type of water filter is the pitcher filter. These are relatively inexpensive to buy and easy to use. One made by a reputable manufacturer should improve taste, make water smell clean and fresh, and reduce chlorine, lead, mercury, and sediment in the water. But you will have to read the literature on it to be sure you are getting all these benefits, as some pitcher products do not provide this level of quality in their product.

FILTRATION SYSTEMS

There is a bewildering range of water filters designed to provide filtered water on tap. Some of them are installed under the sink and work through a separate drinking-water tap placed next to the existing taps. Other systems treat all the domestic water coming into the house from the main supply, filtering the water for washing, cooking, and drinking.

These systems use a whole range of different methods, such as simple filtration, resins, deionization, distillation, and reverse osmosis. Some are better at removing one type of chemical than others, and your choice may depend to some extent on the main pollutants in your water. Generally speaking, though, the following methods are the best at removing overall levels of *Chemical Calories* from your water.

DISTILLATION

This is an effective way to remove *Chemical Calories*, but it is very slow and energy consuming because the water has to be heated up and then cooled. This method is impractical for most people, because it can take up to six hours to produce four liters of water. This kind of system is better suited to producing drinking water, but larger models can be obtained for offices or bigger buildings.

FILTRATION

This is a less expensive and more practical method of removing pollutants. The water flows through a filter, which removes particles that are too large to pass through. Although most manufacturers claim that the filter removes 98 percent of bacteria, chlorine, metals, and pesticides, the amount of chemicals removed really depends on the size and the type of filter used. As many of the pesticide particles can be very small, they may not be caught by the filter. Also, the active part of the filter tends to last for about six months to a year before it needs to be changed. If this does not happen on time, the filter will lose its usefulness. Make sure you buy from a reputable company.

The advantages of this system are that it is relatively quick and efficient, and you can filter large amounts of water straight off the main supply in "real time," making it well suited for a total household supply.

REVERSE OSMOSIS

This method works like a filter: Water is passed through a very fine membrane by applying pressure on one side of the membrane so that the water comes through the other side. Manufacturers claim that this method is very effective in removing between 80 and 98 percent of total dissolved solids, with different minerals having different reduction rates.

One last word on the subject of water filters: The more effective the filter, the more *Chemical Calories* it will remove. However, in removing the harmful chemicals, it will also remove some of the beneficial minerals from drinking water. As water is an important source of certain minerals in our diet, you should make sure that you also take the mineral supplements recommended in Chapter 15.

How Pure Water Helps You Lose Weight

Once you have gotten your *Chemical Calorie*–free water, you should drink lots of it. We know that drinking lots of water can positively help enhance weight loss in several different ways, including:

- Flushing toxins out in sweat and urine.
- Enhancing energy levels by sustaining hydration.
- Burning higher numbers of conventional calories.
- Reducing water retention.

By drinking lots of water, you will be enhancing your body's natural ability to rid itself of *Chemical Calories* in your sweat and urine. And the more you drink, the more you will flush out your system. About eight glasses of pure water a day is ideal to expel toxins.

You might not realize it, but our bodies are largely made up of water: 75 percent if you are an adult. In order to work properly, all these tissues need to be fully hydrated, as even a tiny 2 percent loss in the water surrounding the cells will mean a 20 percent fall in your energy level.[7] This will reduce the amount of energy you can expend and therefore reduce your ability to lose weight.

Before I go any further, when I say the body needs water, I don't mean tea, coffee, fizzy drinks, or alcohol. Herbal tea is fine, as is fruit juice, but all the other drinks mentioned act as diuretics, forcing water out of the body. Thus, for every alcoholic drink you consume, you will lose the same volume of water. It is best to cut out these drinks, but if you can't resist them, do make sure that you drink an extra glass of water for each of these "diuretic drinks" you take in.

Chemical Calories, Water, and Weight

By making the effort to reduce your daily intake of *Chemical Calories* from water, you will be helping yourself lose weight by allowing your *Slimming System* to function more smoothly. A pure water supply will also help you lose weight in another way. As well as reducing the rate at which the body burns off energy, many pollutants can cause swelling and edema by actively reducing levels of the body's natural diuretic hormone, vasopressin anti-diuretic hormone (ADH). The less chemical damage the body incurs, the higher the level of ADH and the less excess fluid your body will carry.

Finally, I found an interesting fact in an academic paper that made a lot of sense to me. It showed that the simple act of drinking water actually speeds up the metabolic rate. This is probably caused by the body's need to heat itself up after drinking a relatively cool liquid. So by drinking cool pure water, you can actually increase the amount of calories you burn off as well as help your *Slimming System* get rid of more weight.[8]

So now we have talked about how to reduce our exposure to *Chemical Calories* from food and water. In the next two chapters, I will deal with the other ways we are exposed to *Chemical Calories*: in our homes and in the environment. The bottom line is that once you have tackled all the main sources of *Chemical Calories* in your life, you will be well on the way to achieving the body of your dreams and keeping it.

However, as our major source of persistent fattening chemicals is our food, you may choose to bypass the next two chapters temporarily and go straight to Chapter 13: Repair and Revitalize Your Natural *Slimming System*, and return to them after you have finished reading about the diet. Whatever you decide to do, put a water filter on your shopping list, pour yourself a glass of water, and read on!

11

Chemical Calories Lurk All Around You: Identifying *Chemical Calories* in Your Home and Environment

By now you will have realized that you are playing by a whole new set of dieting rules, but to succeed you will have to pace yourself. It will take time to process all this new information and then make the changes necessary to create a lifestyle low in *Chemical Calories*. By taking one step at a time, everything will suddenly become less daunting and more doable.

I have already made a number of suggestions about the way in which you can lower the level of *Chemical Calories* in both your water and your food, so try not to be fazed by all the additional information in these next two chapters. You really don't have to do everything at once to achieve weight loss, and you certainly don't have do everything I recommend in this and the next chapter to successfully lose weight.

As the greatest number of persistent *Chemical Calories* will come from your diet, lowering your intake of *Chemical Calories* from food and drink should be your No. 1 priority. A substantial amount of weight loss can be achieved by dietary and supplement changes alone.

One thing you may discover is that as your daily intake of *Chemical Calories* is reduced, your body's ability to reduce its lifelong burden of stored *Chemical Calories* will markedly increase. This is because your detoxification system is no longer forced to deal with the daily onslaught of *Chemical Calories* it was regularly exposed to and can, perhaps for the first time, start to remove these built-up stores and in the process restore your ability to lose weight.

Time and time again, once people experience the incredible slimming benefits for themselves, they actively look for more and more ways to cut out *Chemical Calories* from their lives. This is why I have given you so much information at once: not so you can change everything right now but so you can address different areas when the time is right for you.

The fact is that we are being exposed to more and more *Chemical Calories* in our lives. We absorb them in large quantities from the cosmetics and cleaners used in our homes, from the sprays we use in our gardens, from contaminated air, public transport, the workplace, and even at the dentist!

The information in this chapter will help you limit your exposure to *Chemical Calories* by flagging the highest nonfood sources of these fattening toxins. In the next chapter, I will tell you how to slash your exposure to the vast majority of these problem areas. So don't fret; there are lots of things that can be done to remedy the situation.

How Nonfood *Chemical Calories* Enter Our Bodies

As you would imagine, you will absorb more *Chemical Calories* by eating residues in contaminated foods than by, say, walking past a synthetic toy. Nevertheless, the levels of airborne *Chemical Calories* produced by certain kinds of synthetic substances are significant and real. We are exposed to them all the time.

Some synthetic substances are volatile and evaporate into the air. Others "out-gas," which means that they emit gases that contain *Chemical Calories*. Out-gassing is usually more common in newer objects, which is why carpets and other new furnishings seem to emit a strong odor in the first few weeks and months, after which it becomes less noticeable.

The warmer the environment, the more synthetic substances will out-gas even if they are years old. When you smell the characteristic smell of new carpets or a new car, the chemicals will not just have activated the smelling sensors in your nose, they will also have entered your lungs and from there moved directly into your bloodstream as *Chemical Calories*. And there they will remain until processed by your liver.

Chemical Calories can also readily enter your body through your skin, triggered by the simple act of walking barefoot on treated carpets, by wearing clothes made of synthetic cloth, or by using chemically loaded cosmetics.

Although we are exposed to a generally smaller amount of chemicals through our skin and lungs, these can in fact be just as toxic to our *Slimming System* as those we eat in food (if not more so). Although they will be detoxified to a certain extent in the skin, in bypassing the gut they have effectively avoided all the powerful acids and enzymes that we use in our gut to break down and neutralize chemicals in food.

How Toxic Is Your Home?

Chances are that if you did not build your house yourself or know the people who lived in it previously, it will be very hard to assess how contaminated it is with *Chemical Calories*. Unless the previous owners were known for their environment-friendly ways, it is likely that the products used in the house will have been "conventional" ones, which may have been heavily treated with chemicals.

To some extent, the age of the house will also determine which sorts of chemicals were used. Thirty or forty years ago, carpets and wood were treated with very persistent chemicals such as organochlorines. As a result, unless you have the paperwork detailing what has been used in your house, you may need some expert help.

If you really want to find out the extent to which your house is contaminated with chemicals, you can call in an environmental house doctor. This is exactly what I did to discover how contaminated my house was and to see whether there were any particular problem areas. Samples of household air were collected over twenty-four hours, in addition to bottles of tap water. These were then sent off for analysis.

Fortunately, my house appeared to be relatively uncontaminated, which was a great relief, particularly for my young family. As a matter of fact, the largest amount of chemicals detected were plant-based citrus chemicals from the low-toxicity cleaning products that I used. I have since changed the cleaning products I use, of course, to products that are biodegradable and safely reenter our environment.

The main drawback of this type of investigation of your house is the cost, as the more things you test, the more expensive it becomes. I did it because I live in a very old house and I have only been here for a few years. I wanted to know about any problem areas so that I could deal with them. While the tests are useful, they are definitely not essential. And even if you do consult an environmental house doctor, you still need to find out where the contaminating chemicals are, so you can take positive action.

The rest of this chapter is targeted at identifying the areas of our lives (including the home and the workplace) where we are now exposed to potentially high levels of *Chemical Calories*. Owing to the sheer diversity of chemicals found in different products, it is virtually impossible to be specific about the chemicals in your own home or workplace. However, there are some chemicals that turn up again and again in similar situations. At the very least, the following information should alert you to most of the potential *Chemical Calorie* hot spots that now exist.

What Lurks in the Average Room?

The main sources of *Chemical Calories* in any room stem from the use of the following groups of substances. Unfortunately, they are now used in far more places than most of us could imagine. The four worst offenders are:

- Pesticides
- Synthetics
- Fire retardants
- Solvents

As you can imagine, building materials or furnishings that incorporate these offenders can be potentially loaded with *Chemical Calories*. Because of this, the average room can have many potential hot spots.

A prime example is interior wood that has been treated with preservatives. Think about it: If you have wood treated to prevent woodworm or dry rot, the treatment will be guaranteed for a certain number of years. What this really translates to is that the pesticides inside the wood will be present and active in sufficiently high doses for all those years and will also contaminate the surrounding air and dust.

Dry rot, along with other infestations, can strike fear into the heart of the homeowner, but fortunately there are now natural alternatives available both for providing preventive treatment and for dealing with existing fungal or insect damage problems.

Another fact to consider concerning the woodwork in modern houses is that fiberboard or chipboard tends to be more commonly used nowadays than solid wood. Unfortunately, these can cause a problem from their mixture of adhesives and solvents, which out-gas fumes into the air.

Generally, anything treated with fire retardants (chemicals that slow down the rate of burning) can also be high in *Chemical Calories,* particularly if the extremely persistent chemicals known as polybrominated biphenyls (PBBs) have been used.

Another major source of *Chemical Calories* is certain kinds of synthetic materials, particularly since they are not just used in obvious places such as PVC window frames but are also used in cement, glues, and adhesives. As a result, all these products will potentially out-gas *Chemical Calories* into the air.

One further hot spot is the electric wiring of older houses, for which the organochlorines known as PCBs may have been used as insulation. Unfortunately, PCBs can contaminate the air quite significantly, and in some cases old electric wiring in a house can account for up to one third of the inhabitants' daily PCB exposure.[1]

FLOORING

You may be surprised to discover that a natural product such as wool carpet can often contain more *Chemical Calories* than some synthetic carpets. This is because the manufacturers may have used pesticides to mothproof the wool. The carpet backing of wool and synthetic carpets alike, and even the underlay, all contain *Chemical Calories* from the solvents used in their man-ufacture.

If the carpets have been in place for a long time, the overall amount of toxic fumes will have been significantly reduced. However, many old car-pets made in the mid-'80s were manufactured using longer-acting and per-sistent organochlorine pesticides such as lindane, which are loaded with *Chemical Calories*.

Other "fattening" forms of flooring include vinyl flooring. Again, this re-leases the greatest amount of fumes into the air during the first few months after being laid. Wood and laminated flooring can also introduce *Chemical Calories* if glue or underlay is used, and so can the synthetic-based wood sealants used to give your wooden floor that beautiful shiny polished look.

WALL COVERINGS

Wall coverings also contribute their share of *Chemical Calories* to the air in-side your house. As a general rule, any product that contains vinyl is partic-ularly likely to be high in *Chemical Calories*.

Paint is one of the worst offenders, as it can contain a whole variety of different chemicals, such as solvents, and synthetic colors.

Wallpaper, especially if it is intended for kitchens or bathrooms, can of-ten contain chemicals that will give off gas. In addition, the paste used to apply wallpaper to the walls can contain fungicides.

And while ceramic tiles are fine, the adhesives and grouting used when applying them to the walls can be home to a whole cornucopia of chemi-cals—as I discovered when looking at a can of the stuff just recently.

SOFT FURNISHINGS AND FABRICS

Soft furnishings and curtain fabrics can add a great deal to the attractive-ness of a room; unfortunately they can also add significantly to the toxic chemical cocktail. This is because the law requires that the fabrics used on furniture should pass certain standards of fire resistance.

This can entail the addition of a number of flame-retardant chemicals, many of which can be particularly high in *Chemical Calories,* to slow down the speed at which a product will burn.[2] The level of *Chemical Calories* will be even higher if the furniture is also padded with flame-retardant foam.

I am not telling you that you should choose fabrics without fire retardants; I am just giving you the facts so that you can make an informed decision, weighing all the potential risks in light of your individual situation. The problem with buying furniture in particular is that you can't tell the level of contamination just by looking at the product, and the labels rarely help. Sometimes the information is in the form of coded messages that seem positive and are commonly used as selling points.

Look for information revealing that the product has been heavily treated. If, for example, it is guaranteed to be mothproof or fireproof, you will know that a whole lot of potentially toxic and fattening chemicals have been added; however, it will then be up to you to choose whether you would rather have the qualities that these chemicals bestow or fewer *Chemical Calories.*

What Lurks in the Bathroom?

The typical bathroom can be a relative minefield of *Chemical Calories.* You may not realize it, but behind the hype, many beauty products are far from natural. In fact, many are stuffed with synthetic chemicals. Consequently, the simple act of taking a bath with your favorite scented bath products can increase your *Chemical Calorie* loading. Afterward, as you generously cover your skin with your favorite moisturizing cream, you could be adding even more! So unless you find a reputable natural-product manufacturer that tests its products for high-level safety and nontoxicity, what you are using now may be surprisingly unhealthy for you.

We are constantly told how one product will give us shiny, healthy hair and that another will stop our skin from aging. Whether or not these claims are true, one thing is increasingly clear: More and more personal care products—many brands of hair sprays, nail polishes, perfumes, hair mousse, and a whole range of cosmetics—contain significant levels of *Chemical Calories.* Surfactants (cleaning compounds commonly derived from petroleum) are found in detergents, bubble bath, and shampoos. Again, finding a reputable manufacturer will make all the difference to your *Chemical Calorie* load.

Synthetic preservatives are yet another source of *Chemical Calories.* Most toiletries and cosmetics contain some sort of preservative that will add to their *Chemical Calorie* content. Scientists know that our bodies can absorb much of what we put on our skin. For example, Dr. Philippa Darbre of Reading University, England, has found that lipid-soluble chemicals such as organochlorines (PCBs) readily penetrate skin, then enter the body's circulation. This makes products containing lipid-soluble toxic chemicals a potentially significant source of *Chemical Calories* if we apply them directly to our bodies.[3] Keep in mind that product makers that manufacture high-quality products without using unsafe ingredients such as preservatives do exist.

The other main source of *Chemical Calories* in your bathroom is likely to be your medicine cabinet. I am not talking about prescription drugs here, and I am certainly not encouraging anyone who is ill to stop taking his or her medication. The products that I want to warn you about are the "medicated" shampoos specifically designed for head infestations such as nits, and head and crab lice (but not dandruff). These may contain powerful insecticides, such as organophosphates, and in some states lindane as well, which are extremely toxic as well as high in *Chemical Calories.* And when you put them directly on your skin, a proportion of the chemicals can be absorbed straight into your body. Your doctor, pharmacist, or alternative health-care specialist may be able to recommend alternatives such as fine-tooth combing and natural remedies, which are just as effective as these potentially highly toxic medicated formulas, if not more so.

What Lurks in the Kitchen?

I think you will agree with me that I have already exposed the hiding places of most of the *Chemical Calories* in the kitchen. But what I haven't dealt with is the cleaning closet, which you will shortly discover is a real *Chemical Calorie* hot spot! By taking a look at their labels, you will discover that many household products are quite frankly downright scary in the number of toxic chemicals they contain. Needless to say, quite a few products are particularly high in *Chemical Calories* from the concoction of preservatives, perfumes, solvents, detergents, surfactants, and emulsifiers that they possess. While I don't suggest you put down all your cleaning tools, I would advise you to use more natural alternatives, about which there are a number of suggestions in the next chapter.

Many kitchens also contain common household pesticides. You may not think you use pesticides, but in reality very few houses are without them. You probably have them in the form of fly killers, ant poisons, mosquito sprays, rodent controls, insect repellent, and all the many forms of pet products such as flea powder, flea sprays, and shampoos for fleas, lice, and mange.

All these products tend to be high in *Chemical Calories,* but the good news is that, as with cleaning products, there are plenty of alternatives. After all, these problems have been around for a very long time, long before synthetic chemicals were ever created.

What Lurks in the Bedroom?

The bedroom is a particularly important room, as most of us spend more than one third of our lives there. Consequently, if any room needs to be free of *Chemical Calories,* this should be the one. Let's start with the bed.

Because of current fire regulations, most mattresses are now covered with fire retardants, which we now know can act as a major source of contamination. But the mattress is not alone here: The coverings and pillows can also be treated with fire retardants, adding further to the overall *Chemical Calorie* loading of the bed. As mentioned above, if you have a relatively high fire-risk factor, for example, if you smoke or have an open fire in your bedroom, it will be best to keep the flame-retardant items but minimize the *Chemical Calorie* effect by using the methods described in the next chapter.

Apart from the bed, your wardrobe tends to be the other major source of *Chemical Calories.* Some will originate from clothes that contain chemicals, such as synthetic leather or waterproof garments. Other clothes will have *Chemical Calories* added in the manufacturing process—look out for labels that say "fire resistant," "easy care," or "easy iron."

You can even be responsible for adding *Chemical Calories* yourself if you dry-clean your clothes (because of the solvents used in cleaning) or if you use certain chemically treated mothballs to prevent insect damage.

The Children's Playroom

Go into any toy shop and you will be greeted by a strong smell of chemicals wafting through the air. Take a good look around you and you will soon see why. The vast majority of new toys are made from highly toxic PVC and a whole range of other chemically treated materials that have replaced more traditional materials such as wood.

Although some countries have withdrawn chemical-laden toys that are designed to be chewed during teething, there appear to be no restrictions on PVC's use in other children's products. I am not suggesting for one moment that you throw all the kids' toys out—first, this is not necessary, and second, it might just trigger a rebellion (I know it would in our household anyway!)—but just that you should make sure they are stored properly and that the rooms they are stored in are well ventilated.

Other children's products high in *Chemical Calories* include glues used in all kinds of art and model making, paints, felt-tips, play mats, protective sheeting, bath books, laminated board books, and soft toys.

The Garden Shed and Garage

The garden shed, or anywhere that you store building and gardening materials, can be a huge source of *Chemical Calories*. Old cans of paint and varnish are highly volatile and can contain a large number of synthetic chemicals such as surfactants, lead, styrenes, and solvents. These areas can also contain toxic glues and adhesives for use all over the house as well as wood preservatives for garden fences and furniture. On a warm day, you can really smell these toxic substances, because they will evaporate into the air more quickly.

Garages are not particularly healthy places on the whole, as they tend to contain lots of *Chemical Calorie*–rich sources such as oil, gasoline, solvents, and detergents, which tend to evaporate. On top of this, oil, gasoline, and diesel fuel are also adulterated with a whole range of additives including lead, organophosphates, synthetics, detergents, and a whole lot more highly toxic and fattening chemicals.

The problems get worse if your garage is connected to your house and the overall ventilation is poor, as the chances are that the fumes will waft straight into your home. And if you park your car in an integral garage, then by starting up the engine in this confined space, you are likely to send yet more fumes into your living space.

Let's now move onward and outward to the garden. Far from being a natural and relaxing environment, the modern garden is becoming a toxic battlefield! *Chemical Calories* abound in the ordinary garden shed: pesticides to kill insects and weed killers to remove unwanted plants from your paths, flower beds, or lawn.

These chemicals are bad enough in the garden, but did you know that lawn herbicides, for example, can be tracked indoors on your or your children's shoes and on your pets' paws, and can contaminate carpets for a long time? What's more, dogs that roll around on herbicide-treated lawns tend to be more prone to getting a certain type of cancer (non-Hodgkins lymphoma).[4]

These facts are starting to be more widely appreciated, and many gardening books and programs now recommend organic methods to control weeds and pests. Any changes you make in this direction will make your garden and home a safer place too.

What Lurks in the Workplace?

As you can imagine, different occupations will vary greatly in their exposure to *Chemical Calories*. Certain factory workers, painters and decorators, hairdressers, and mechanics tend to have relatively high exposure. In most cases, the majority of this contamination is through their lungs and skin. But they are not the only ones at risk, for even office workers can be regularly exposed to chemicals in stationery or newly laid carpets, or in the cleaning solutions used on office furniture. On top of this, some buildings are regularly sprayed with insecticides to prevent infestations, which could increase employees' exposure to *Chemical Calories* quite dramatically.

Chemical Calories at the Dentist

Advances in dentistry and dental awareness mean that we tend to keep our teeth for much longer than our ancestors did. In order to achieve this, dentists now use a whole range of substances to patch up or replace broken teeth. The problem is that any substance on our teeth is likely to be ground up and swallowed with the rest of our food.

Recently, I had to embark on a long course of treatment because of breaking one of my teeth on a piece of organic homemade popcorn—yes, strange coincidence, isn't it? This experience really opened my eyes to the substances dentists now use routinely. For instance, I discovered that most of the materials used by dentists as temporary fillings or sealants contain mixtures of chemicals. The materials used to get dental impressions also contain chemicals that can leach into your system, and amalgam mercury fillings contain heavy metals.

Even if you choose the safer option of repairing teeth with porcelain, the repair is usually made with synthetic materials, unless you request otherwise. Even false teeth are made with synthetics! All these materials will potentially leach *Chemical Calories* into your mouth. The amount of chemicals seems small, but because repair materials are constantly wearing away in your mouth and being ingested, the level of contamination from many of these interventions can actually be measured in your blood.

In the *Canadian Dental Association Journal*, Dr. M. Levy suggests that more research should be carried out into the potential health effects of certain dental materials, such as dental amalgam. And he also suggests that in the meantime, more of an effort should be put into preserving healthy teeth, and that the restorative dental materials in current practice should be used more judiciously.[5]

While I definitely don't want to stop you from going to the dentist, I urge you to find out from your dentist what your options are and then choose the safest treatment. (I opted for the porcelain repair.) And if you need an alternative to amalgam fillings, gold fillings are thought to be much less toxic, because gold is a relatively inert metal.

Chemical Calories Are Everywhere

Finally, *Chemical Calories* bombard us from all directions as we walk, shop, and take part in local activities. But now you know where the problems are and are ready to do something about them. In the next chapter, I will help you deal with them by telling you about the easy ways in which you can significantly lower the *Chemical Calorie* content of your home. It won't take too long before you realize that it is possible to make a significant difference without too much expense or upheaval. So don't be too depressed, because there really is light ahead!

12

Beating the *Chemical Calorie*: Reducing Your Overall Exposure

The beauty of reducing the amount of *Chemical Calories* in your home is that by lowering your overall exposure to them, you will be making real advances in preventing further damage to your *Slimming System*. In time, this is what will help you achieve and maintain your ideal weight, so it's worth making a real effort to discover how it can be done.

Since I started to cut down on *Chemical Calories* in my food and home, I no longer have any fear of the scales. My *Slimming System* is now strong enough to maintain my weight on its own. In fact, despite not actively dieting, and still having some of my favorite foods daily, I am continuing to lose weight—slowly, I admit, but the trend is still downward. I am delighted, as I now have a figure that I am very happy with and that requires very little effort to maintain.

Now it's your turn to discover my secret!

Where to Begin—Air Your Air

As I previously mentioned, the first thing you need to do is pace yourself. It is simply not possible to create a *Chemical Calorie*–free environment overnight, and in any case it is not necessary to endure the time, cost, and inconvenience of ripping everything out and starting all over again. There are lots of simple ways to significantly reduce the *Chemical Calories* in your home that will require very little effort.

For example, as a large number of *Chemical Calories* in your home will be airborne, the quickest way to get rid of them is simply to open the windows. Try to make sure that you open windows at the front and back of the house, as this will increase the flow of air. This is particularly important in new houses, as many of them are now hermetically sealed. Ventilating the house for just half an hour can really make all the difference.

Even if you live in a city, indoor air still tends to be far more polluted than city air, so it is still a good idea to allow some ventilation. Of course, if you live next to a very busy road, it would be wise to close the windows during peak-hour traffic. If the outside air is exceptionally polluted, you could always consider investing in an air filter, which filters out pollutants, many of which will contain *Chemical Calories* from exhaust fumes.

Another way of reducing *Chemical Calories* is by filling your home with plants. It has been found that spider plants, Boston ferns, elephant-ear philodendron, English ivy, and aloe vera appear to be particularly efficient "air filters" and are very good at removing solvents from the atmosphere.[1]

Get Rid of Household Pesticides

One of the really positive things you can do to lower the *Chemical Calorie* content of your home is to get rid of all your pesticides. By that I mean your fly sprays, insect repellents, flea powders, flea shampoos, head lice shampoos, weed killers, ant and slug killers, and all other types of home and garden pesticides. But don't put them down the sink, where they will poison the water supply; dispose of them responsibly. Many local authorities provide safe disposal for these toxic chemicals at town dumps and waste-recycling centers, so if you clear out these chemicals from your kitchen or garden shed, there is a place where they can and should be disposed of safely.

Next, you will need to find alternative treatments. For example, if your dog has fleas, then rather than spray the whole house with toxic chemicals, you could use an herbal shampoo or spray and buy an herbal flea collar, which contains natural repellents such as pennyroyal or eucalyptus oils. There are even herbal flea powders to use on carpets and furnishings. They usually contain pyrethrum (a plant extract) or borax.

Throughout the rest of the house, you can use citrus oils to repel flies. Try spraying the room with a solution of essential citrus oils and water. You can eliminate cockroaches by mixing equal parts of baking soda and powdered sugar. Spread this mixture where they congregate and repeat every one to two weeks until they are gone.

To eradicate ants, you can use mint. (They can't stand it.) Mix one cup of water with two teaspoons of essential oil of peppermint, and spray the mixture wherever the ants come in: on windowsills, countertops, and along baseboards.

There are so many natural remedies; unfortunately, I don't have the space to cover them all here. I suggest you consult a reputable natural-products company that you know you can trust. You will find that because of health worries from modern-day pesticides, many of the long-forgotten traditional ways of pest control are being rediscovered and are coming back into favor.

Alternative Cleaning Solutions

The vast majority of domestic cleaning products contain a cornucopia of toxic and fattening chemicals, so the best thing is to try to find alternatives. Cleaning a home doesn't require complex ingredients. You'll find plenty of alternative highly effective cleaning products made by reputable natural-product makers. In fact, you will find a whole section on this in Chapter 19.

If there are particular products for which you really can't find a replacement, it's a good idea to seal them up in an airtight container such as an old cookie tin. This will significantly reduce the amount of vapor they release into the air, which will otherwise end up in your lungs.

Keeping *Chemical Calories* Out of Clothes and Fabrics

In order to keep the *Chemical Calorie* content as low as possible in clothes and fabrics, you have three priorities. The first is to try to buy clothes and fabrics made of natural fibers (provided there are no residual pesticides on the latter). The second, if you consider yourself or the recipient of the clothing to be at low risk from fire, is to avoid fabrics that have been treated with flame-retardant chemicals. And the third is to check whether the fabric has been chemically treated to be "easy care."

Synthetic fabrics will off-gas *Chemical Calories*. For most people, switching to natural fibers is not really a problem, since the selection is pretty extensive, but you still need to be careful about chemical finishes. The ideal solution is to buy organic fabrics.

While sometimes hard to find, natural organic untreated fabrics, clothes, and other goods come from a range of sources that includes hemp, cotton, wool, silk, and linen. The market for organic fabrics is growing rapidly because of environmental concerns about the vast amounts of pesticides used in growing cotton. It's sad but true that pesticides for cotton growers have been estimated at a stunning third of the entire worldwide production of pesticides.[2] If you buy organic fabrics, you have a guarantee that no added pesticide residues or chemicals will be found on them, and you also know that they haven't contributed to the contamination of the land. Indeed, many people who wear them are convinced that organic fabrics are not only softer but also stronger.

The main disadvantages are their limited colors and designs and generally higher price. However, things are changing on the color front, and more organic companies are looking into the use of vegetable dyes or low-impact dyeing methods. Low-impact dyeing uses synthetic dyes but minimizes the use of synthetic chemicals in processing the fibers. As with everything, pester power is the key to making these products more widely available. The more people who ask for chemical-free clothes, the more likely companies are to introduce new lines.

Even if you can't get organic clothes, you should ask whether the clothes have been treated with flame retardants, as many big companies are starting to cut down on the routine treatment of clothes with these chemicals, particularly those for babies and toddlers.

While on the subject of clothes and fabrics—if you dry-clean clothes, curtains, and other items, they will be covered in a solvent that contains lots of *Chemical Calories*. Either hang your clothes out to air in a well-ventilated place for a few days after dry cleaning, or, best of all, try to find a dry cleaner who uses steam instead of solvents.

One last point: It's generally best to use one of the growing number of environmentally friendly detergents that are available.

The Low–*Chemical Calorie* Garden

Once you have chucked out all your herbicides, weed killers, insect sprays, and other noxious substances (responsibly, of course), you will have significantly lowered your exposure to *Chemical Calories*. The next step will take a little longer, as you need to discover new techniques to discourage weeds and pests naturally.

Since agriculture played such a vital role long before chemicals were invented, there is already a mountain of information on traditional practices. Much of it has been ignored for years, but a growing number of farmers are reviving older methods to farm their land and raise their animals organically. If you take your gardening seriously, there are now lots of books available on organic horticultural techniques. Another good source of information can be found at the website www.organicgardening.com.

To keep down the number of pests in your vegetable garden, you can achieve a lot with a technique known as *companion planting*. Some pests identify crops by scent, so a neighboring crop with a powerful scent (such as onions) will confuse them. Even if you don't grow vegetables and want to preserve your roses, planting chives around your roses will not only protect them from disease but also somewhat surprisingly enhance their perfume too.

Another technique is to encourage your allies, the predators that feed on aphids and other pests. A pesticide cannot recognize the difference between good and bad bugs and just kills the lot. But by leaving piles of wood, stones, or leaves undisturbed over winter, where many ladybugs and other predators hibernate, you can tip the balance in favor of the predators and use them to reduce the number of aphids in your garden. Did you know that one ladybug eats many thousands of aphids in a lifetime?

Birds are also excellent predators, though they tend to eat your soft fruit too! I have just created a flower garden near my vegetable patch and filled one area with flowers to encourage pollinators and another area with flowers that produce seed heads for birds. I am also exceedingly fortunate to have an organic vegetable garden that provides us with mountains of food throughout the year. To help us achieve this, we make our own compost from our kitchen household waste.

I have to say that few pleasures in life can compare with eating freshly picked fruit and vegetables brimming with flavor and bursting with oodles of slimming nutrients.

Avoiding *Chemical Calories* in Your Environment

You can do quite a lot to lower the level of *Chemical Calories* in your home, but there is relatively little you can do about air pollution outside. If you are planning to move, the best areas to live in are those away from large factories, big cities, major roadways, and areas of intensive horticulture.

There are also some things you can do to reduce your exposure where you now reside. If your house is surrounded by fields that are sprayed regularly, make sure that the farmer tells you when he intends to spray so that you can stay indoors and keep your windows closed. If you have children, going to parks may be a regular event for you. Try to find out if your local park uses lots of pesticides to control weeds. If they do, you should stay clear of the areas where they spray, and stay away altogether while the spraying is going on. The same holds true if you live in an agricultural area. Never walk through a field just after or during spraying.

Even when you are driving in your car, you can be exposed to large amounts of *Chemical Calories* from the other cars on the road. The best answer may be to get an air filter for your car. Also try to stay more than four car lengths behind the car in front of you, as this gives the exhaust some time to disperse before you drive through it—not to mention giving you more time to react in case of an accident ahead!

The Next Step Forward

Now you know how to lower your exposure to *Chemical Calories* in many different areas of your life, and by gradually implementing these changes you will be well on your way to achieving the goal of permanent weight loss. However, it will still take your body time to rid itself of all the *Chemical Calories* that it has built up over the years.

Most people will prefer to see quicker results, and the good news is that this process can be speeded as well as greatly enhanced by using supplements, foods, diet, and exercise. In Part Three, I will tell you how the proper use of these methods can not only significantly enhance the functioning of your natural *Slimming System* but can also accelerate the rate at which *Chemical Calories* are removed from your body. Unlike most diet books, which are simply based on methods that starve you of calories, the whole emphasis here is feeding and protecting your natural *Slimming System*. The next chapter is brimming with all the information you need to revitalize your natural *Slimming System,* simply by feeding it the foods and supplements it needs.

Part Three

DETOXIFY AND
LOSE WEIGHT

13

Repair and Revitalize Your Natural *Slimming System*

By now you know a great deal about avoiding exposure to *Chemical Calories*. While this aspect is important for the success of the program, it is only part of the overall strategy to lose weight. Now we need to turn to the next major task, which is to optimize your own natural *Slimming System*.

If your *Slimming System* were in perfect working order, it would take on the work of dieting for you, adjusting your appetite and metabolism so that your body would lose weight without any conscious effort. In other words, by rebuilding your natural *Slimming System*, you will be working with your body and not continually battling against it to lose weight and keep it off, effectively releasing yourself from a lifetime of dieting and deprivation.

So what does it take to rebuild the *Slimming System*? Fortunately, most of the work can be done by a combination of the right foods and supplements. The chances are that you got into this predicament because your body, overloaded with *Chemical Calories,* badly lacks many of the essential slimming nutrients that it needs because of the increased demands made on it. To help pull your *Slimming System* out of intensive care and back to full health, I will go through all the foods and nutrients that it needs in order to resume its proper function. Then watch those excess pounds just melt away!

145

How Certain Fats Can Make You Slim

Fats have unfortunately gotten a very bad name and are often seen as the enemy of dieters. But in fact the right kinds of fats are absolutely essential in achieving weight loss, as without them our *Slimming System* would fail to work properly.

Not all fats are the same. Your diet actually contains two different kinds of fats: Most of them will be saturated (bad) fats, typically animal fats, but only a few will be the essential (good) fats, typically fish oils or fats from nuts and seeds. Saturated fats are not essential to our diet, since we can make them ourselves. In fact, most people's diets contain far too many saturated fats.

Worlds apart are the essential fats: polyunsaturated and monounsaturated fats that are quite essential to our diet. This is because our bodies cannot manufacture their own supply and therefore are totally reliant on our eating foods that contain them. They are also vital to the smooth working of the *Slimming System*. To put it bluntly, without them we would simply not be able to lose weight efficiently.

Although the very idea that fats can make us lose weight is counterintuitive, healthful fats help us achieve weight loss in the following ways:

- Massively increasing the rate at which we burn up our body fat stores.[1]
- Increasing the levels of energy we can produce from food. (The more energy we create, the fewer calories we store as fats.)[2]
- Stabilizing blood sugar levels, thereby reducing sugar cravings (and preventing the development of diabetes).
- Boosting the levels of slimming hormones, in particular the hormones that suppress our appetite for fats (catecholamines).
- Raising our body's sensitivity to slimming hormones, thereby speeding up the rate at which calories are burned.
- Improving our ability to retain slimming vitamins and minerals in our bodies.[3]
- Suppressing free-radical production and so preventing damage

to our *Slimming Systems* (particularly in the more crucial high-fat-containing parts).[4]

If you are not getting enough essential fats, your ability to lose weight will greatly pick up if you start consuming them. Despite the fact that most people's diets contain a substantial chunk of fat (typically, 40 percent of the total calories), little of this is essential fat. The hard reality is that, unless you are making a special effort to include these fats in your diet, chances are that you will be deficient in them—disastrous news for your ability to lose weight!

The Importance of These Essential Omega-3 and Omega-6 Fats

So why are these essential fats so important? The reason is based on how we lived many thousands of years ago, when humanity was in its infancy. At that time, we were a shore-dwelling people and tended to eat large quantities of fish as well as to scavenge for nuts and seeds. As all these foods contained large amounts of omega-3 and omega-6 oils, which are the essential fats that possess these slimming actions, our bodies adapted to use these fats extensively—and we still need them just as much today.[5]

However, over the years our diet has changed dramatically: Our intake of nuts and fish has decreased, and our food has become more processed. As a direct consequence, the quantity of essential fats in our diet has fallen.

Modern-day living also conspires in other ways to lower the level of fatty acids in our diet. Heat not only rapidly destroys the slimming benefits of essential fats but also transforms them into harmful substances known as trans-fats, which prevent us from absorbing any of the remaining essential fatty acids. Olive oil, however, is safe for use in cooking, as it contains fats that don't tend to form trans-fats. Butter also does not tend to form trans-fats, but butter is a saturated fat.

So by eating fried foods such as chips, you could actually be reducing the absorption of the essential fatty acids that you do manage to eat in your diet. Other types of food processing also produce these trans-fats, for example, the process of turning vegetable oils into margarine (hydrogenation).

Making a bad situation worse, few processed foods and ready-made meals contain any beneficial essential fat. This is because beneficial fats tend to go bad more quickly, reducing the shelf life of foods that contain them. So you can see that because of our changing lifestyles and habits, most of our bodies are now crying out to be fed more essential fats.

How to Remedy the Situation

Omega-3 fats are the ones that you are most likely to be deficient in, particularly since they are easily damaged in their natural form. They also appear to play a more important role in lowering our weight. Many people already take omega-3 supplements in the form of fish oils. However, because some of them have been found to be polluted with *Chemical Calories*,[6] it is best to buy them from reputable natural-product sources that acknowledge there is a potential problem and therefore actively source fish that are clean and test the oils regularly.

Organic flax, one of the earliest crops known to be cultivated, is another rich source of omega-3 oils whose importance has been acknowledged for years. (Its name in Latin means to "the much needed.") You can buy it in liquid form (also known as linseed oil) to take orally or in capsules if you find the taste unpleasant (for the recommended dose, see Chapter 15).

While they are both excellent sources of omega-3 fats, for some people fish oils have a major advantage over flax oils. This is because fish oils possess omega-3 fats in a form the body can use readily. The problem with flax oil is that our bodies must convert it before we can use it. Although most people can convert flax oils into a usable form, some individuals cannot because they do not have enough nutrients to power the conversion. In addition, a small number of people simply have a genetic inability to process these oils.

Another sensible way to boost your intake of omega-3 fats is by consuming them, as they are found in cold-water fish, in seeds such as flax and pumpkin, and in certain nuts such as walnuts. To a lesser extent, they can also be found in wild meats such as venison and in some other meats, particularly if they are organic. This is because the higher the animal's diet is in omega-3 fats, the higher the level found in the meat.

Omega-6 fats are found more widely, and on the whole we tend to have larger amounts of these fats in our diet because more foods contain them. For example, most vegetable oils contain far higher levels of omega-6 oils than omega-3 oils, and they are also found in flax oil, seeds, fish oils, nuts, and meats.

Consequently, there is not such a great need to supplement omega-6 fats, but to ensure you are getting enough on this program, I advise that you do take evening primrose oil or the alternative listed in Chapter 15. The message is: Eat more essential oils and less saturated fat, and you will be more likely to lose weight.

The Role of Carbohydrates in the *Slimming System*

Recently, a whole new generation of diet books has virtually demonized carbohydrates, blaming them for weight gain and a host of other problems. Certainly excessive carbohydrates, particularly sugary selections, can cause weight gain, but moderate levels of the right kind of carbohydrates are essential for the smooth running of the *Slimming System*. For example, be sure you keep eating healthful portions of beans, fruits and vegetables, and healthy grain products. They are the body's basic fuel for energy, and without them a whole range of body functions begins to shut down. So let's find out a bit more about what carbohydrates are and where they can be found.

Carbohydrates play an absolutely vital role in powering the *Slimming System,* because they:

- Ensure that your muscles are packed with readily accessible sugar stores, so you have plenty of energy to power exercise.
- Increase energy levels and so encourage exercise.
- Greatly raise your metabolic rate, as they strongly stimulate the sympathetic nervous system, thereby promoting the release of the slimming hormones catecholamines, epinephrine, and nor-

epinephrine. This results in converting up to 20 percent of the original energy value (calories) of all the carbohydrates you eat into heat that is then easily lost.

- Suppress the appetite for more carbohydrates, preventing potential bingeing.

Although the system was designed to work smoothly, the presence of *Chemical Calories* has changed all this by damaging the ways in which the body metabolizes carbohydrates.

I have experienced this myself. For years before I took supplements or ate organic foods, my own ability to control my sugar levels was appalling. If I didn't eat something every two or three hours, my blood sugar would take a dive. I would get into a real state. My concentration would go first, then I would get very sweaty. And if I didn't eat something right away, I would get even worse. My husband quickly came to recognize the signs; he could spot a crisis in the making long before I could and made sure I had something to eat immediately. Now, since I have lowered my exposure to chemicals and started taking supplements, I really don't have this problem at all, because my body now seems to be able to regulate my blood sugar on its own.

I was therefore not too surprised when, during my examination of the relevant research, I discovered that chemicals appear to damage carbohydrate metabolism in a number of different ways.

- The appetite for carbohydrate increases, caused by a number of factors such as damage to a whole range of hormones that control the appetite for sugar.[7]
- Chemicals interfere with the process of converting glucose into usable energy. In other words, the body is less able to use carbohydrates.[8]
- Dieting exacerbates this damage. People, particularly women, tend to eat need more sugary foods rather than starchy foods after dieting.[9]

The damage caused by *Chemical Calories* could explain why overweight people appear to have a reduced ability to break down carbohydrates. When overweight people, who generally as a group tend to have higher levels of chemicals in their bodies, go on a fast, they use approximately half as much carbohydrate as lean people use.[10] Even when they are given readily usable glucose, overweight people still tend to draw on fats for energy rather than on carbohydrates.

This diminished ability to metabolize carbohydrates fully also explains why there has been a rash of very-low-carbohydrate diets on the market. But while the idea seems like a good one on the surface, there are many problems associated with the exclusion of virtually all carbohydrates from the diet.

The Pros and Cons of Low-Carbohydrate Diets

By cutting right back on carbohydrates, you will certainly reduce the amount of excess carbohydrates that can be converted to weight. You will also lower the levels of insulin, and this increases mobilization of the body-fat stores. Superficially, this seems like a very plausible idea and will probably achieve good temporary weight loss.

However, the presence of fattening chemicals is another significant cause of weight gain, and cutting carbohydrates out of the diet will definitely not treat this. In truth, there are many disadvantages to a very-low-carbohydrate diet, and they include the following:

- Increased absorption of pesticides, as pesticides are far more readily absorbed from high-fat foods than from high-carbohydrate foods.[11]
- Reduced ability to metabolize toxic chemicals, as this process needs carbohydrates.[12]
- Reduced stimulation of the sympathetic nervous system, which results in reduced fat burning.
- Huge carbohydrate cravings caused by low blood sugar, which will trigger the release of hormones.
- Shrinkage of lean muscle, as your body needs to break down muscle to produce readily usable sugars.
- Reduced levels of slimming micronutrients usually found in carbohydrate-rich foods such as fruit and vegetables.

151

- Increased release of fat-soluble toxins, as more fats are mobilized.
- High risk of arteriosclerosis, because high levels of mobilized fats and cholesterol in the blood, in combination with prolonged low insulin levels, are known to increase the likelihood of heart disease and strokes.

So while eating too many carbohydrates can make us fatter, too few will have the same effect in the long term and the potential to cause more serious damage. The ideal is to eat carbohydrates in moderation and to choose complex carbohydrates, as they release their sugars over several hours rather than in one massive rush. And the simple sugars that you do eat should be mainly in the form of fruit.

You have to realize that until your chemical loading is tackled, you will still crave sweet foods. Though, as the levels of *Chemical Calories* drop, your ability to handle carbohydrates, like mine, will greatly improve. And as well as significantly reducing your sugar cravings, fewer *Chemical Calories* will also mean that you'll start burning up carbohydrates more efficiently.

The Proteins That Keep You Slim

Virtually all aspects of the *Slimming System* are controlled in some way by substances or structures containing protein. So an upset in protein metabolism or a shortage in any particular protein can result in damage to any one of the numerous mechanisms vital to controlling our body weight. So which types of proteins are we talking about?

Let's begin with the basics: A protein is a large, complex molecule that is made up of units known as *amino acids*. There are approximately twenty-nine different amino acids in the body, of which eight are "essential," meaning the body cannot manufacture them and must get them from food and supplements.

Despite their name, many of the "nonessential" amino acids are absolutely vital for the smooth functioning of the body, but we can usually manufacture them ourselves if we do not get enough from other sources. So how do they control our weight?

In brief, proteins are used by the *Slimming System* to:

- Form the structure of the most important slimming hormones.
- Speed up the metabolism (protein-rich foods can lift the metabolic rate to 30 percent above normal for three to twelve hours).
- Facilitate energy production.
- Build muscles so that we can burn off body fat during exercise.

How Chemicals Damage Proteins

The problem with toxic chemicals is that they appear to damage virtually every aspect of the way our body handles, absorbs, and creates proteins as well as to increase the rate at which they are lost from the body.[13] They even directly damage the proteins themselves.

So although we may think we are eating enough proteins, chemical damage means that our bodies can fail to extract and use the proteins they need to allow our *Slimming System* to work properly. This chemical damage is caused in the following ways:

- By lowering levels of amino acids that we specifically need to create our slimming hormones (catecholamines and thyroid hormones).[14]
- By damaging the way our body responds to slimming hormones.
- By upsetting our body's natural rhythm so that billions of carefully timed sequences are thrown out of sync, making the whole metabolic system less effective. This systemic upset will also severely reduce the body's ability to burn off excess fat.[15]
- Hindering the creation of all types of body proteins, including those proteins essential to energy production and calorie burning, such as body muscle.[16]

What You Can Do About It

We all need to include a moderate and balanced amount of protein in our diet to keep the *Slimming System* in peak working order. So where can we find the proteins we need? Most people assume that we get most of our proteins from meat, dairy products, and eggs. While these are very rich sources, they are not the only ones; a whole range of fruit, vegetables, nuts, and beans also contains proteins. OK, although these sources can be less rich, in combination they are still well able to supply the protein needs of the *Slimming System*. Soy protein is the most biologically complete protein there is and can be fixed in absolutely delicious ways. Soy is high in protein, low in fat, naturally cholesterol- and lactose-free, and provides essential amino acids that the body needs but cannot produce itself.

The presence of toxic chemicals makes it more difficult for the body to get and create all the proteins it needs from food alone, so it is a good idea to supplement key slimming proteins in the diet. There are four basic protein supplements that I believe everyone needs.

The first is *methionine,* because it is the amino acid most damaged by chemicals. It plays one of the most essential roles in promoting energy metabolism, so it is particularly important to ensure that you get enough.

The next is *glutathione.* Glutathione plays a main role in chemical detoxification and therefore is always in great demand to keep your *Slimming System* functioning properly.

Third is *tyrosine,* which forms the base structure for the most important slimming hormones of all, the catecholamines and the thyroid hormones. Many of us tend to be short of this vitally important protein because we are unable to create enough of it ourselves as a result of chemical damage. It is better to take tyrosine supplements in the morning, as they will help boost your energy levels.

And finally, we need more *serotonin,* which powerfully suppresses the appetite. Low levels of serotonin will result in food cravings and binge eating. As serotonin is also readily damaged by the presence of chemicals, it is definitely worthwhile to supplement it. Ideally, you should take serotonin in the form of its precursor, L-5 hydroxytryptophan, before you go to sleep, as it can make you drowsy.

The good news is, as your loading of *Chemical Calories* falls, your ability to use and create new proteins will increase and your need for these supplements will be reduced. For most people whose bodies are loaded with *Chemical Calories* right now, protein supplements will be of great benefit in helping to get their *Slimming Systems* back into shape. A healthy *Slimming System* will soon be followed by a shapely body!

Vitamins and Minerals

By now you will already have heard quite a lot about our need for vitamins and minerals. You will also have realized that they play a crucial role in our *Slimming Systems* and that our need for them is greatly increased by chemicals. But before I go on, let's start with some basic information. What exactly are vitamins and minerals, and where can you find them?

Vitamins and minerals are naturally occurring substances that are essential to normal growth and nutrition. The body cannot synthesize them, so we must get them from our diet or from supplements. Because we need only very small amounts, they are commonly described as micronutrients. Although they are often referred to as a duo, their structures differ greatly.

Vitamins are complex substances that are made by plants, tend to be fragile, and are easily destroyed by heat. Minerals are substances found in the earth's crust that are absorbed by plants, which use them for their own growth. Although these micronutrients have no caloric value as such, they are vital components of a healthy diet because they are used as catalysts for most of the processes needed to sustain life: They enhance growth and energy production, quicken our metabolism, allow detoxification to take place, activate our immune systems, facilitate reproduction, promote longevity, and among other things, they also help to keep us slim.

How Vitamins Are Essential in Powering the *Slimming System*

Vitamins and minerals play a pivotal role in weight control. Because of their role as catalysts in speeding up the millions of reactions taking place daily in our bodies, they allow us to convert foodstuffs and body fat into energy. So, to a large extent, they actually determine our ability to burn calories.

For example, vitamin A is essential in the burning of fat and its conversion to heat. But it is also vital in the processing of chemicals. So if the body is exposed to larger levels of chemicals, there will be less vitamin A left to burn fat and thus encourage weight gain. As the presence of some chemicals can actually halve the body's store of vitamins, this effect simply cannot be ignored.

But it is not just vitamin A that is important; many other vitamins and minerals play an equally important role in powering our *Slimming System* and ridding our body of *Chemical Calories*.[17] This is why in this book I have often described these micronutrients as slimming, because that is often just what they do.

Why We Need More and More Vitamins

In affluent countries such as the United States, it is difficult to imagine that vitamin and mineral deficiencies exist on a broad scale, because food is so readily available. However, because of the falling levels of micronutrients in our foods and our increased intake of processed foods, growing numbers of Americans are simply not getting enough micronutrients from their diets. The population groups at highest risk are women, the elderly, adolescents, low-income groups, ethnic minorities, infants, and children.[18]

These deficiencies are exacerbated by the presence of chemicals in the world, as they have sent our need for the vitamins and minerals essential to detoxifying chemicals skyrocketing. So it seems that while our need for nutrients has never been higher, our intake is unable to keep pace with our body's increasing demands.

This shortfall of vitamins has most probably massively reduced our ability to keep off excess weight. It has also likely increased the vulnerability of our *Slimming System* to chemical damage. Bad news for us girls, as women appear to be particularly vulnerable because we tend to eat less food. This reduces even further the opportunity to extract all the micronutrients we now need. Perhaps it also helps to explain why women are gaining twice as much weight as men every year.

Optimizing Your Nutrient Levels

The micronutrients that play a crucial role in powering the *Slimming System* include vitamins A, B_1 (thiamine), B_2 (riboflavin), B_6 (pyridoxine), C, E, coenzyme Q_{10}, and the minerals magnesium and zinc, among others. (The lists of supplements required for the diet and for long-term use can be found in Chapter 15.)

Even if you cannot get all the micronutrients you need just from your food, it is still a good idea to eat foods that are high in slimming micronutrients, such as uncooked vegetables, salads, and fruits. The highest levels of slimming nutrients appear to be found in organic produce, and the fresher the produce the better, since levels of vitamins will fall during storage and plummet during cooking. So it's hard to beat the amount of slimming nutrients in a fresh salad of organic fruits and vegetables.

As well as their micronutrient content, unprocessed raw foods also appear to contain a whole range of other nutrients, known as *phytonutrients,* which also seem to have some role in enhancing our *Slimming System.*

In addition to eating a certain amount of fresh raw organic produce every day, it is now essential to supplement your diet with tablets containing high levels of vitamins and minerals to ensure the smooth running of your *Slimming System.* Because this requires a whole range of micronutrients, it is best to take a multivitamin and mineral supplement. You can top with larger individual doses of certain micronutrients if necessary. However, if you take one or two large doses of individual vitamins or minerals without a good general multivitamin, they will be far less effective and possibly unbalance your *Slimming System.*

So we now need supplements, not just at levels aimed at preventing deficiencies but at levels that will optimize the *Slimming System.* By ensuring that your rate of vitamin and mineral supplementation is sufficient, you will be helping your body to slim. Fortunately, as much of the harm done by low levels of micronutrients can be reversed, it is never too late to start!

So now we know what to feed our *Slimming System* to optimize its efficiency. Next, we need to deal with the *Chemical Calories* already stored in our bodies that continually damage our *Slimming System,* particularly when we actively cut down on food.

Please understand this: No longer do you have to be stuck with a body full of *Chemical Calories* for life, because it is now possible to remove them from your body safely. Once this is achieved, your *Slimming System* will be boosted to a new level of efficiency, thereby converting your dream of permanent weight loss into reality.

14

Shed Your Body Stores
of *Chemical Calories*

Now we know how to cut out *Chemical Calories* from our food, homes, water, and environment. Nevertheless, before we can fully benefit from these efforts, we need to get rid of the massive amounts of *Chemical Calories* that have been building up within our bodies throughout our lives.

Fortunately for us, there are safe ways in which we can remove the most persistent and fattening *Chemical Calories*. In this chapter, I will tell you how to shed this buildup safely. By doing so you will revitalize your *Slimming System* and reap health and energy-giving benefits that will enable you to get the utmost enjoyment out of your new slimmer and fitter body.

The Real Baddies

Knowing your enemy is the first step in defeating it, so it is time to talk about the most fattening *Chemical Calories* of all, the persistent fat-soluble organochlorines. The simple fact is that we have no efficient natural way of breaking them down and removing them from our bodies. They are very stable, highly soluble in fat, and tend to "take up residence" in the body's fat stores.

Because toxic chemicals are stored in body fat, the myth that they are relatively safe has arisen. But body fat is not just inert or stuck there for life. Over the course of each two to three weeks, all the body-fat stores are broken down, circulate in the bloodstream, and then are re-created. As it is virtually impossible to separate these chemicals from fat, wherever these fats go, so too will the organochlorines.

Conventional Dieting Can Make You Fatter

I think most of us who have ever been on a diet know from experience that while we might achieve a temporary weight loss, after a few months not only will we have regained all the weight we lost, but the chances are that we also will weigh more than we did before we even started. What's worse, most of this extra weight tends to be fat. Why does this happen?

It all stems from the fact that when people go on a conventional diet, they eat less food. Our bodies then urgently need to produce energy from somewhere, and as one of the most readily available sources of energy is body fat, it is used as an energy source. If the energy demands are too great, however, our body fats will be broken up far too rapidly, resulting in large amounts of stored toxins, which have accumulated over the years, being released into the bloodstream. These toxins then circulate and cause increased damage throughout the body.[1] To make matters worse, because many of the most essential parts of our *Slimming System,* such as our hormone-producing glands and our brains, have such a good blood supply as well as a high fat content, they are exceedingly vulnerable to damage from these highly fat-soluble chemicals.

Common ways in which we experience this poisoning in the short term are nausea, fatigue, headaches, and general malaise.[2] This may explain why people can feel unwell or get headaches during the first few days of a diet.

The weight problems come from the damage done to the *Slimming System* following this exposure. The greater the damage, the higher your weight set point is likely to become, which means that your weight will stabilize at a higher level. This tendency to damage the *Slimming System* is one of the main reasons conventional diets tend to cause weight gain in the long term.

Why Fasting Can Also Be Dangerous

It is not just dieting that can be dangerous; the more extreme forms of food restriction, such as fasting, can be too. Over the centuries, different cultures and religions have developed their own techniques to help the body detoxify itself, and until fairly recently they were very successful. Most of these techniques depend on fasting, drinking only water, or spending a few days drinking fruit and vegetable juices. Some methods incorporate particular herbs or foods.

In a world without chemical loading, fasting was a spiritual experience as well as a bodily purge. Now that our bodies store such harmful chemicals, however, these techniques can be extremely dangerous. I find this very sad, particularly since fasting has been practiced for many years and can have great religious importance.

The risks of fasting can be worse than those of dieting alone, as the level of food restriction is more extreme: When people fast, they usually totally deprive their bodies of food rather than just cut back. The resulting level of toxins mobilized can be up to 300 percent above the normal blood levels, a level far greater than that brought on by dieting alone, and this has the potential to cause greater damage to our *Slimming System*. (If you need to fast for religious reasons, there are ways in which it can be made safer, and these will be discussed later, in Chapter 16.)

The Harmful Nature of Dieting— My Painful Story

A few months after my second son was born, I was absolutely desperate to lose weight and get into my old clothes again. The very sight of my maternity clothes was almost too much to bear.

As I was extremely busy with two young and very demanding boys, I fell back on a diet based on a very low carbohydrate intake that I had used before. However, I quickly discovered that it was totally unsuitable for me, as it proved far too restrictive and led to huge cravings for carbohydrates coupled with an almost continual headache. When the headache finally wore off, I experienced general muscular aches and fatigue for months. I gave up on the diet, but in the meantime I felt so ill that I sometimes had to stay in bed when I most wanted to get out and enjoy my family.

This is definitely not what you need at one of the most enjoyable but stressful periods in your life. I know now that I experienced firsthand many of the toxic effects that stored chemicals have on our bodies when they are mobilized. Although I have never felt better than I do now, I certainly never want to experience that illness again, as I felt I lost a chunk of my life in the process.

How These Persistent *Chemical Calories* Can Be Removed from Our Bodies

However, there is a bright side. After personally experiencing the effects of *Chemical Calories*, I wholeheartedly embraced the fact that they were a real problem and was spurred on to understand exactly how and why the problem occurs. Once you understand how it happens, it becomes possible to find a workable solution.

There are actually many different ways in which we can shed these *Chemical Calories* from our bodies. Curiously, many of the early studies were performed not with humans but with cows and other farm animals that had been contaminated with organochlorines from their feed. Farmers had to either remove the chemicals from the animals or not sell them for human consumption and suffer financial loss.

Tests showed that animals given extra rations of specific vitamins and minerals were much more able to rid their bodies of these chemicals. In some cases, the rate of excretion of certain organochlorines more than doubled.[3] While this technique was obviously safe and very useful, it was still relatively slow. Another, more efficient method needed to be found.

It soon became apparent that one of the best techniques was to take advantage of the natural recycling of fats in the gut. As fat is broken down, it is released into the blood, taking with it its collection of organochlorines. Some of the fats are then secreted from the blood into the gut in the gastric juices and travel through the gut until they are absorbed back into the blood again in the small intestine. These reabsorbed fats are then put back into the body stores. This journey forms a "fat cycle" that begins at the fat stores, travels round the gut, and then returns to the fat stores. Fortunately, it also creates a window of opportunity to remove these chemicals while they are in the gut.[4]

This window of opportunity can be utilized by oral administration of substances that bind in the gut not just to the recycling fats but also to the pesticides and other fat-loving synthetic chemicals. Once they are firmly bound to these "carriers," the pesticides will not be reabsorbed further down the gut but instead will be carried out of the body with other waste products.[5]

This method of feeding "binding" substances to highly contaminated animals to make them "safe" to eat has actually been highly effective in ridding animals of persistent *Chemical Calories*. The main substance used in previous research studies was charcoal. Indeed, one study showed that charcoal was so effective in reducing the level of the very fattening chemical DDT (an organochlorine) that it also resulted in the animal losing fat.[6] In the eyes of the farmer, any weight loss effect was not likely to be appreciated, and this was commented on in the study as being a potential problem. Looking at it from a dieter's point of view, it is fantastic news, because it indicates that by ridding your body of persistent *Chemical Calories*, it is possible to lose fat as well.

The conclusions from these findings are clear. The extensive contamination of our bodies with *Chemical Calories* means that the whole way we diet now needs to change. Any attempt to lose fat must now include a detox program. If we don't deal with the very high levels of toxins released, ordinary methods of dieting that use food restriction alone will not only damage the *Slimming System* and make us fatter but also could potentially ruin good health in the process.

Anyone who is really serious about losing weight needs to adapt the way he or she diets to our more polluted environment. Only by doing this will we ever be successful in losing weight permanently. So how do we do it? To answer this, we need to know a bit more about the ways in which our bodies detoxify.

The Trials of Detoxing

The ability to detoxify will vary greatly from one individual to another. The extent to which *Chemical Calories* build up in a person's fat and other body parts depends not only on how much they have been exposed but also on how efficient their bodies are in eliminating these chemicals.

Genetic makeup is one very important factor. Some people will be better at detoxifying than others because they were born with more powerful enzyme systems, which are better able to break down chemicals. This could result in some family members being less able than others to detoxify and being far more vulnerable than others to chemical-related problems such as excess weight and to chemical-related illnesses such as cancers and allergies.

As well as differences in inherited resistance, what you eat will also largely determine how good your natural detoxification system is. If you have a highly processed diet deficient in many essential nutrients, then the chances are that your detox system will be struggling.

In our caveman days, we probably used to consume many times more vitamins and minerals in our foods than we do now because of the large amounts of raw foods that were eaten. Despite the wider range of foods available today, the amount of raw nutrient-rich food in our diets has dramatically fallen, so we are functioning on levels of vitamins and minerals far lower than they have ever been. When we diet, as the amount of food we eat falls and our diets become more and more deficient in essential nutrients, we end up having substantially fewer resources available for detoxification, which accelerates the buildup of toxins over time.

If We Understand the Problem,
We Can Turn This Situation Around

Luckily, unlike our genetic makeup, which we cannot change, this is a situation that we can actually do something really positive about. The simple act of taking certain nutrient supplements can enable our detoxification systems to work to their best ability and therefore boost the rate at which these toxins are eliminated from our bodies.

Another problem arises from the fact that much of our diet is so highly processed. As well as being low in slimming nutrients, these processed foods will also reduce our natural ability to detoxify because when they break down, they will increase our body's acidity levels. An acidic environment significantly slows down the rate at which our detoxification enzymes can work. That being the case, an increased level of processed foods will make detoxification just that much more difficult. Other acid-producing foods include meat and dairy products and diet sodas. On the other hand, alkaline-producing foods such as fruit and vegetables or certain supplements will optimize our ability to detoxify.[7]

As well as genetic makeup, our age also plays an important part in how vulnerable we are to chemical damage and in our ability to detoxify. Those who are very young or very old are the most vulnerable. Young immune systems are not fully developed and so are less able to kick out chemicals. Consequently, they can be damaged by far lower levels of chemicals than those needed to cause damage in adults.[8]

At the other end of the age scale, the ability to detoxify will fall significantly with age due to an overall reduction in efficiency of the detoxification systems.[9] The good news is that you can boost the efficiency of your detoxification system at any age and, as a result, lose weight. So how do we go about doing that?

How to Shed *Chemical Calories* Safely

The most important way to start is to minimize any further buildup of *Chemical Calories* in your body. This can be achieved by eating organic foods or foods low in *Chemical Calories* and by cutting down your exposure to *Chemical Calories* in your household and environment (see Chapters 7 to 12). By not continually adding to your load, you will be giving your body a chance to deal with its chemical backlog.

Next, you will need to help your body use its natural detoxification system to the fullest by giving it all the nutrients it needs to perform optimally (see below). Then you need to start actively ridding your body of the most persistent *Chemical Calorie* contaminates by providing your body with extra help in the form of "binding" substances that you can then excrete naturally.

All About Binding Substances

Although charcoal is a useful binder, a more widely available substance is soluble fiber. This is not the kind of fiber that tends to be known as roughage but fiber that can form a gellike consistency when mixed with water. Soluble fiber includes substances such as psyllium husks, the fiber commonly found in beans and oats, and other naturally occurring plant fiber such as pectin, found in many fruits. All these binding substances can be readily bought as supplements from quality natural-products companies, and I will explain later how you should use them.

These binders are invaluable tools for removing the most persistent *Chemical Calories* from your body. They have a powerful ability to bind themselves to dangerous toxins that you can then excrete safely.[10]

I will just mention here that not only can these substances bind the most persistent *Chemical Calories*, they also can bind some of the essential slimming nutrients that we need.[11] So while taking any of these detoxers, you will need to ensure that you are getting a generous amount of vitamins and minerals in the form of supplements. Ideally, take the vitamins and minerals at least half an hour or preferably an hour after soluble fiber. This should ensure that you get enough nutrients to optimize your *Slimming System*.

Furthermore, binding substances such as soluble fiber can be so effective at binding chemicals that they could potentially bind with any medications you are taking, thereby reducing their effect. So check with your doctor before taking these particular substances if you are on prescribed medications, particularly the contraceptive pill or thyroid hormone-replacement treatment, which could possibly be rendered ineffective.

Once you have slowed down your intake of *Chemical Calories* and boosted your ability to rid yourself of existing ones using the right nutritional supplements, you will be well on your way in tackling any excess weight. With this new way of using natural substances to absorb mobilized *Chemical Calories* in the body, it will now become much safer to diet.

In fact, if performed with a mild degree of food restriction and a more intensive exercise regime, the rate at which you will shed *Chemical Calories* from your body will be accelerated. As long as you follow the advice carefully, by combining a mild food-restrictive diet with "binding" substances in the form of supplements and foods, you will create an extremely effective way of eliminating *Chemical Calories* from your body.

The presence of these binding substances will also keep the level of blood-borne *Chemical Calories* low, reducing any potential damage to your *Slimming System*. As a result, the toxins and your excess weight should gradually disappear together, leaving you lighter, healthier, and reenergized. By adopting this system, we can adapt the way we lose weight to the problems of the twenty-first century.

What We Need to Do
to Shed *Chemical Calories*

So, in review, the five-step process for shedding even the most persistent *Chemical Calories* is as follows:

1. Keep your chemical load down. The less exposure your body has to *Chemical Calories*, the better it will be able to deal with processing the *Chemical Calories* it already has.
2. Feed your detoxification system with nutrients. The right nutri-

ents will help you shed *Chemical Calories* faster and protect your natural *Slimming System* from toxic damage.

3. Take soluble fiber to draw the most persistent *Chemical Calories* out of the gut, as these very fattening chemicals are not easily removed by any other means.
4. Use mild food restriction to mobilize toxins stored in body fat.
5. Exercise to mobilize fat stores and enhance your detoxification processes.

Supplements Are Essential for Enhancing Detoxification

Many supplements will be needed, some in larger quantities than usual, to maximize the rate at which we can break down these *Chemical Calories*. One of the most important organs in which this breakdown occurs is the liver, so to achieve maximum rates of detoxification, we need to ensure that our liver gets enough nutrients.

Our liver needs a whole range of vitamins, minerals, amino acids, essential fatty acids, and sufficient supplies of carbohydrate to effectively power, permit, or speed up the thousands of different reactions that are taking place in your body around the clock. The more stress placed on the liver by higher levels of *Chemical Calories,* the more nutrients the liver will need to do its job.

But it is not just the liver that needs feeding: The very presence of *Chemical Calories* in our bodies will create another need for nutrients because of the increased production of free radicals. Many *Chemical Calories* trigger the release of free radicals into our tissues. So what are free radicals?

Free Radicals

A free radical is a particle with an attitude.[12] It knocks around the tissue in which it finds itself and tries to destroy all the structures present. The body can soak up these tissue-wreckers, but it needs to use some of its precious supply of antioxidants (such as vitamins C and E) to limit the damage. This results in lower levels of antioxidants available to power our *Slimming System*.

The drain that *Chemical Calories* make on many of our essential nutrients doesn't stop there, as these substances can in themselves reduce our ability to absorb nutrients from our food by damaging the complex mechanisms involved. What's worse, they can even increase the rate at which many of these slimming nutrients are excreted from our bodies.[13] In other words, stored *Chemical Calories* leave us with even fewer nutrients for detoxification and repair, so the more damage we have done in the past, the more nutrients we now need to fix our systems.

But before you rush out to buy your supplements, you need to know what can happen so you will be prepared: Some people who start to take vitamin and mineral supplements may temporarily feel mildly worse for the first few weeks before they feel better. But for the first time in years, the body will actually have sufficient resources to start dealing with the massive buildup of stored chemicals.

This unexpected side effect is quite real—I experienced it myself. When I mentioned it to a knowledgeable professor friend of mine, he said it was because I was detoxing. I must admit that at the time I was very skeptical, but since then I have seen the same thing happen to many people when they start taking supplements. The temporary ill effects are most probably caused by the increased mobilization of chemicals that are in the process of being broken down.

Don't be disheartened if this affects you. On the contrary, you should realize that it is happening because the supplements are having the desired effect. Keep going, and this phase will soon wear off. You will soon be rewarded with a higher level of health, which is of course accompanied by permanent weight loss.

Feed Your Detox System

Many multivitamins that you can buy from local shops or many big discounters are thought to be insufficient for optimizing your ability to detoxify. This is because the recommended levels are the minimum amount you need to prevent vitamin deficiencies or the products are not sufficiently bioavailable to be absorbed into your bloodstream.

It is getting clearer that our need for certain vitamins has increased because they are the ones that are excreted more rapidly from our bodies by chemicals or are used up in larger quantities when we process toxins. More recent studies have shown that we now have an increased need for vitamins A, C, and E at levels far above those stated in the Recommended Dietary Allowance (RDA).[14] So to boost your ability to kick out *Chemical Calories* and prevent any damage to your *Slimming System* in the process, the supplements that you take need to have higher levels of these particular vitamins that tend to get used up more quickly.

If these particular nutrients were really "slimming" vitamins, you might expect those people who are deficient in them to be overweight. Well, several studies have shown this to be absolutely true. In fact, the more overweight a person is, the lower the level of these vitamins will be in their bodies.[15] This is probably related to the fact that overweight people will tend to use these nutrients faster and/or simply don't get enough in their food. These lower levels will then impair the running of their *Slimming Systems*, which will result in weight gain.

So by taking the right supplements, which are readily available, you can easily ensure that you are getting enough nutrients. For the products and doses that I recommend, see Chapter 15.

The Nutrients We Now Need to Enhance Removal of *Chemical Calories*

People concerned about their health typically choose a supplement made out of only vitamins and minerals. The problem is that our need for other nutrients, besides vitamins and minerals, has also increased, due to the presence of *Chemical Calories* and our increasingly processed diets. As many of these other nutrients play a vital role in boosting the functioning of our detoxification and of our *Slimming System*, it is essential to ensure that we get sufficient levels of these other nutrients too. I will now give more detail about what these other substances are and how they can enhance our ability to detoxify.

AMINO ACIDS

As seen earlier, the problem with chemical pollutants is that they damage the way our bodies break down, absorb, use, and manufacture amino acids. This is why people who are damaged by chemicals are frequently deficient in amino acids, despite seemingly adequate levels in their diet.[16]

Certain amino acids are absolutely crucial to our ability to detoxify ourselves of chemical pollutants, particularly the harder-to-shift organochlorines,[17] which include methionine, cysteine, taurine, and glutathione. These can be found in many of the foods listed on the *Slimming System* detoxification diet, but to ensure that you receive optimal levels, you could always also supplement some of them.

LIPID SUPPLEMENTATION

As previously discussed, although eating fats takes some getting used to for people who want to lose weight, the right fats are absolutely essential for successful slimming because they allow your slimming hormones to work fully.

The fats you eat also have a significant effect on the toxicity of chemicals because some fats can alter your ability to break down the chemicals. Diets that are deficient in certain essential fatty acids, such as omega-3 and omega-6, limit our ability to detoxify chemicals.[18] Fish oil or flax oil, for example, will greatly improve your ability to break down *Chemical Calories* and will make them less toxic. Consequently, these fats play a crucial role in powering our detoxification systems. On the other hand, saturated fats, such as animal fats, appear to have no such protective effects.

Our need for these essential fatty acids becomes even greater when we are dieting. High levels of newly mobilized *Chemical Calories* will readily destroy essential fats, possibly because of the increased levels of free radicals that *Chemical Calories* create. This destructive effect could be reflected by the fact that dieting has been associated with a fall in the body's level of omega-3 fatty acids.[19]

To prevent any drop in essential fatty acids, we need to increase our intake of them during times of food restriction. This will prevent any drop in our levels of essential fatty acids just at the time we need them the most. The recommended doses for these highly effective and vital "slimming" fats can be found in Chapter 15.

PH BALANCE

Although most people know about the need for certain nutrients in our diet, very few know that pH is also crucial. The pH balance of your body is the relative level of acidity/alkalinity and is vitally important in enabling the detoxification enzymes to work properly.

Unfortunately, most people's food intake is too high in acid-producing foods (meat, cheese, and diet sodas) and too low in alkaline-forming foods (fruits and, particularly, vegetables). This means that the enzyme systems of most people do not function properly. As a result, their ability to detoxify *Chemical Calories* is seriously reduced. This is why an alkalinization supplement or drink is useful for people who are actively dieting, as it will promote more effective and more rapid removal and processing of *Chemical Calories*.

If you already eat a diet rich in fruit and vegetables, or the very diet presented in this program, you may not need this supplement. If you want to check, you can test your own urine to see whether it is alkaline or acidic by using a piece of litmus paper. If you are already hypertensive (have high blood pressure) or have a renal (kidney) or cardiac (heart) impairment, then you should not take this supplement but should drink vegetable juice instead.

BINDING AGENTS

This is a general name for substances used to draw out toxic *Chemical Calories* from the body. They play an exceptionally important part in my program, because they are among the few substances that can lower the level of virtually all the different types of *Chemical Calories* found in the body.

Soluble fiber is the most popular kind of binding agent. You can buy it in supplement form as psyllium husks or fruit pectins and gums, which are widely available from natural-products companies. It has been estimated that we eat far too little dietary fiber in our daily diet. The average U.S. citizen eats 12 to 17 grams of fiber per day, whereas the American Dietetic Association recommends that the total level of dietary fiber in an adult's diet should be much higher, 20 to 35 grams per day.[20] So you can see that we should eat significantly more fiber than we currently do. And if you are on any medication, check with your doctor first, as these supplements could potentially neutralize or interact with certain medications.

When and how to take these binding agents
A good time to take these substances is immediately after waking up and before breakfast, as your night's fast will have mobilized your fats and increased your blood levels of *Chemical Calories*. They can also be taken with meals throughout the day, especially when following the Body Restoration Plan Diet, as mild food restriction will increase the mobilization of *Chemical Calories*.

As a precautionary measure, however, it is best not to take vitamin and mineral pills at the same time you take binding agents. Also, you should drink plenty of fluid with soluble fiber, in particular with psyllium husks, as they tend to absorb lots of water.

HERBAL REMEDIES

There is a large range of other natural substances that can be used to improve detoxification and can also be used during the detoxification diet. Perhaps the best known is milk thistle, a powerful antioxidant and a great tonic for the liver (see Chapter 15). Other natural detoxers include grape seed, burdock, red clover, fenugreek, echinacea, yellow dock, dandelion root, ginkgo biloba, and gingerroot. Strictly speaking, none of these substances are essential nutrients, but they do seem to improve our ability to detoxify and so could be beneficial.

WATER

It is vitally important to drink filtered water in sufficient quantities to help wash away some of the *Chemical Calories* from the system, particularly if you are mobilizing *Chemical Calories* from your fat by dieting or exercising. I would suggest that an intake of at least eight 8-ounce glasses of water per day is vital, and if you are restricting your food intake, then you should increase this to at least ten to twelve glasses of water every day. Don't forget, if your body becomes mildly dehydrated by just a few percentage points, the level of energy you can produce can drop by 20 percent.

CARBOHYDRATES

Although you might not expect it, carbohydrates appear to be absolutely essential to our ability to detoxify. This is because many of the individual reactions taking place need a certain amount of readily available sugar. Consequently, very-low-carbohydrate diets can actually hinder our body's ability to detoxify, as they effectively starve the detoxification enzymes of the nutrients they need so that they cannot work to their full capacity. As a result, food-restriction diets should always include a certain amount of carbohydrate, and very-low-carbohydrate diets should be avoided.

Use Food Restriction, Exercise, and Other Methods to Enhance Detoxification

If you cut out *Chemical Calories* from your life as well as take all the supplements I have previously mentioned, you will be well on your way to significantly lowering your inner *Chemical Calorie* levels and in turn enhancing your long-term weight loss. This is fine for people who don't have much weight to lose or who don't mind taking a longer time to bring about weight loss. But for those of you who want to speed up this process, there are now several ways in which you can do so safely. All involve approaches that combine taking the above-mentioned supplements and using the following ways of mobilizing body fats.

FOOD RESTRICTION

Severe food restriction, and fasting in particular, can be very toxic, as it greatly increases the level of *Chemical Calories* released into the blood circulation without providing an exit route for them. However, following a mild food-restriction diet with increased levels of vitamins, supplements, and binding agents can be a great way to detoxify and speed up the safe removal of highly toxic and fattening chemicals.

EXERCISE

Exercise, if performed for a long period of time, can create the same effect. This is because extensive periods of exercise will increase the amount of fat burned, which will therefore increase the amount of *Chemical Calories* released. Exercise also has the added bonus of increasing the oxygen supply to the body, which will greatly help the detoxification process.[21]

The best general advice here is to take it steady, and if you are on a food-restriction diet, don't overdo the amount of exercise in the first few weeks. This is because the levels of *Chemical Calories* are likely to be at their highest during the first few days of a food-restriction diet. So it is best not to increase these high levels still further by undertaking excessive periods of exercise. This doesn't mean you should totally stop all forms of exercise—far from it—just that you should initially refrain from undertaking excessively vigorous spells of exercise for hours on end.

One more comment: To get the maximum detoxification value from the exercise you do, you need to be taking the supplements recommended in Chapter 15. This will also ensure that your *Slimming System* is protected from the increased levels of free radicals released by exercise.

HEAT TREATMENT

Taking a sauna or a steam bath has the effect of mobilizing *Chemical Calories*. As with exercise, you can use this method to boost detoxification, particularly if you take the supplements recommended for this program.[22] Remember to keep drinking lots of water though.

I would also recommend body scrubbing or dry-skin brushing, as these will accelerate one of the few natural ways in which the body can rid itself of persistent *Chemical Calories*—the shedding of dead skin cells. Many people also recommend colonic irrigation, but there is a risk of removing good bowel bacteria, so it wouldn't be my first choice for detoxing.

Now that we have dealt with the extremely important subject of how to shift your body's stores of persistent *Chemical Calories* safely, it is time to progress rapidly to the diet itself. By now you will understand that synthetic chemicals have changed the way our bodies work. As a result, all the previous diets that have ignored their effects are not only obsolete but also potentially dangerous. Those who seriously want to shape up will need to bring the way they diet into the twenty-first century. Fortunately, we now have the know-how to achieve this dietary revolution. Read on to discover the exciting new secrets of how to lose weight, not just for a few weeks but for the rest of your life!

15

The Body Restoration
Plan Diet

The Body Restoration Plan Diet has been designed specifically for those who want to lose weight more quickly than they would normally expect to by cutting down on their *Chemical Calorie* intake alone. This is because a period of mild food restriction can accelerate the rate at which *Chemical Calories* can be removed from the body. The aim of the Body Restoration Plan Diet is to provide a safe way to maximize the body's ability to shed its load of *Chemical Calories*. I have also tried to make it a very easy diet to follow, whether you like cooking or prefer to keep food preparation simple.

It is a mildly food-restrictive diet, which means that, unlike many other diets, every day will not be a battle between you and your appetite. It is also designed to give your *Slimming System* the foods it needs to maximize its efficiency: In other words, you will be helping it shift your excess body fat at the fastest rate possible.

From previous experience, I have found that the more rigid the diet, the less likely I have been to stick to it. Because of this, I have kept the rules very flexible. This is a massive advantage, as we all have different preferences and different degrees of access to organic foods, and therefore we need an equally flexible diet that we can follow at work, at home, or eating out.

Principles of the Diet

This diet has four basic principles, which, if followed, will help those pounds slide right off.

1. *Feed the body's detoxification system*
The intention is to provide your body with the resources it needs to detoxify. So the emphasis will be on eating sufficient quantities of the right foods, rather than on just cutting down on food consumption in general. It is also vital that you take the supplements recommended in this chapter.

2. *Eat the right foods*
Your intake of raw foods, particularly vegetables, should be maximized. They boost your ability to detoxify for all the following reasons:

- They contain masses of valuable slimming nutrients.
- They are high in fiber and will act like an internal broom.
- They are alkaline, which aids detoxification.
- They contain enzymes that play an important roles in digestion, reducing the burden on the body to produce its own enzymes for breaking down foods.

3. *Keep* Chemical Calories *low*
It is very important to reduce your exposure to *Chemical Calories* throughout the time you are dieting. This will enable the body to put all its energy into removing persistent chemicals from its fat stores. You should be selecting foods that are known to be low in *Chemical Calories* or those that are prepared in such a way that they become low in *Chemical Calories* (see Chapter 9).

Another way to ensure that your intake of *Chemical Calories* is kept as low as possible is to combine foods potentially high in *Chemical Calories* with a food high in soluble fiber. Beans, lentils and other legumes, oats, and fruits such as apples and oranges will soak up extra *Chemical Calories* from other ingredients so that you absorb fewer *Chemical Calories* into your body.

4. *Mild food restriction*

The aim of this diet is to restrict food mildly rather than dramatically. If fat stores are mobilized too quickly, the body will not be able to detoxify quickly enough to keep pace. So don't expect to lose too many pounds each week. Set your sights at a maximum of 1 to 2 pounds per week or 1 percent of your body weight. If you lose weight much faster than this, you will probably be losing not fat but muscle and water, which definitely won't make you slim in the long run. In addition, the less weight you have to lose, the less dramatic your progress will appear. Just take things according to your own situation.

There are also two other elements of the program that will contribute significantly to the success of all your efforts: exercise and keeping a record of your progress.

Exercise Is Vital!

As you can imagine, exercise is extremely important to help you lose weight and essential to maintaining your new, slimmer self. Did you know that exercise appears to be one of the few ways in which you can actually lower your body's natural weight? And people who keep exercising after they have lost weight are far more successful in keeping it off than people who fail to keep up their activity level. If you want to keep your newfound body, you have to keep working on it!

The Importance of Keeping a Journal

One of the best ways to keep yourself motivated during a weight management program is to keep a close record or journal of the progress you have made. So before you start, find time to weigh and measure yourself, and record it in your journal. These measurements could make a world of difference to your morale for the rest of the program. In addition, you will really kick yourself later if you don't, because you won't be able to see how far you've come!

Daily Journal
DATE: Beginning weight this week:
MORNING DETOXIFIERS Supplements: Food:
NOON Food:
EVENING Supplements: Food:

Water: ❑ ❑ ❑ ❑ ❑ ❑ ❑

EXERCISE
What did you do today?

How long?

WHAT WORKED TODAY?

Who Should Use Food Restriction to Lose Weight?

Adults who are genuinely overweight should use food restriction as part of their weight loss plan. By including a mild food-restrictive element, they can get down to their target weight in a much shorter time. Then, when they are close to their target weight, they can drop the food-restrictive element of the diet and lose the last few remaining pounds just by following the advice on how to maintain weight loss given in Chapter 18.

However, not everyone needs to cut down on food intake to lose weight. If you are just a few pounds heavier than you want to be, you can probably lose them just by following the advice in Chapter 18, which involves taking supplements and adopting a regular exercise routine. These measures will strengthen your *Slimming System* and lower your body weight set point. The main drawback here will be the time it takes to lose those few pounds. If you are happy with your weight but just want to improve your shape and muscle tone, this gentler method is for you.

On the other hand, some people, for example, very young children, pregnant women, or those who are breast-feeding, should not go on a food-restriction diet even if they want to lose weight. Still, eating foods that are low in *Chemical Calories* and naturally high in slimming nutrients and soluble fiber can only be good for you and your baby. If you are pregnant or breast feeding, you should consult your physician before taking supplements.

The good news is that even people who cannot restrict their food intake can follow the other principles of the program, and I will talk more about these issues in Chapter 18.

Starting the Body Restoration Plan Diet

At this point, I have already covered most of the principles behind the Body Restoration Plan Diet. In the remainder of this chapter, I will lead you through the stages of putting the whole program together. The first stage is to buy the supplements and start taking them in the recommended quantities (see below).

As I discuss the necessary supplements, I will suggest some dietary supplement products that I believe are ideal for anyone following the Body Restoration Plan Diet. They are products that I found when I was looking for supplements that contained natural ingredients; had no volatile organic solvents, no preservatives, pesticides, or toxins; and could offer scientifically proven potency and bioavailability. In other words, I was looking for science-based products made by a company with a long-standing reputation for quality and integrity. I found those products made by a company called Shaklee®.

Shaklee and its products fit perfectly with the philosophy on which my Body Restoration Plan Diet is based. The company's mission is to create healthier lives, and they have been developing high-quality natural products for more than forty-six years. Shaklee tests all its ingredients for quality, strength, and purity; they don't do it just once or twice but sample three lots of every new ingredient. On top of that, the company has been known to go right to the actual growing locations to get the finest raw materials. Products are formulated to be highly bioavailable, which means that Shaklee's ingested nutrients are absorbed into the bloodstream and don't just pass through the digestive tract.

To learn where to purchase Shaklee products, you can visit www.shaklee.com or call (800) 742-5533.

After getting your supplements, you should start taking them for at least two weeks before starting the diet. This is vitally important for several reasons:

- It allows you to source all the supplements and get into a routine of taking them at the right times of day. As there are quite a few supplements to take, this will give you one less thing to contend with when you start the diet.
- Your body will have a chance to get rid of some *Chemical Calories* that are easily removed, thereby reducing the burden of detoxification when you start to diet.
- The body's natural *Slimming System* will be strengthened by the supplements and be better able to protect itself from potential damage when the diet starts.

If you already take supplements, but not all those suggested, it is still better to give your body a week to prepare itself properly. Don't forget, in this time you will also be learning the lifelong habits you need to stay slim as well as improving your ability to lose weight, so it really is worth getting into the routine.

Supplements for Dieters

The easiest and best way to get the vitamins and supplements you need is to purchase top-quality products that offer a combination of all the necessary supplements. That way, you won't have to take as great a number of pills and capsules but will be able to limit your regimen to just a few to swallow. Below is a specific list of vitamins, minerals, and other supplements you can take to enhance your weight loss while restricting your food intake. You will need to take a combination of supplements, because no single supplement will contain the exact levels of all the nutrients you need. Your best option is to take a high-quality, high-potency multivitamin and mineral formula, flaxseed oil and/or pesticide-free fish oil, and soluble fiber, and then add specific extra supplements to bring your nutrient intake as close as possible to the figures below.

Essential Supplements	Total Daily Amount*
Vitamin A (preformed or beta-carotene)	5,000–10,000 IU[†]
Vitamin C	500–2,000 mg
Vitamin D	400–600 IU
Vitamin E	400–800 IU
Vitamin K	80 mcg
Thiamin[‡]	10–25 mg
Riboflavin[‡]	10–25 mg
Niacin[‡]	25–50 mg
Vitamin B_6[‡]	25–100 mg
Folic acid[‡]	400 mcg
Vitamin B_{12}[‡]	10–50 mcg
Biotin[‡]	300 mcg
Pantothenic Acid[‡]	25–50mg
Calcium	500–1,000 mg
Phosphorus	350–1,000 mg
Iodine	150 mcg
Magnesium	200–400mg
Zinc	15–30mg
Selenium	135–200 mcg
Copper	2 mg
Manganese	3.5 mg
Chromium	400–800 mcg
Molybdenum	160 mcg
Iron[§]	18 mg
Choline[§§]	25–100 mg
Coenzyme Q_{10}	30 mg

*NB: IU = international units; mcg = micrograms; mg = milligrams; 1,000 mcg = 1 mg
[†]If pregnant or trying to conceive, do not exceed 10,000 IU of preformed vitamin A each day.
[‡]Higher levels of B vitamins may be appropriate and safe to take for the purpose of lowering serum homocysteine, preventing birth defects, and/or protecting against age-related cognitive decline.
[§]Adult men and postmenopausal women do not need supplemental iron unless treating iron-deficiency anemia.
[§§]Soy lecithin supplements are a good source of supplemental choline.

The Body Restoration Plan

The levels of recommended supplements are based on the accumulation of a very extensive amount of published research on the benefits of dietary supplementation over the past few decades in both the United Kingdom and United States. In particular, I relied on the research of Dr. E. J. Cheraskin, who over a fifteen-year period established the Optimal Nutrient Allowances for vitamins in more than 10,000 Americans.[1] It is also based on Dr. W. Rea's work in treating more than 20,000 chemically sensitive patients at the Environmental Health Center, based in Dallas, Texas.[2] And finally it takes into account some of the values recommended by the U.K. Department of Health.[3]

A good foundation product for the Body Restoration Plan Diet is *Shaklee Basics®*, which provides the essential vitamins, critical minerals, and

ESSENTIAL FATS	TOTAL DAILY AMOUNT

Omega-3 essential fats
    Noncontaminated fish oil taken
      with meals*
    or
    Linseed oil/flaxseed oil
 and
 Omega-6 essential fats
    Gamma linoleic acid†
	500 mg EPA and 900 mg total
	 omega-3 fatty acids
	
	 5–15 g (approx. 1 to 3 teaspoons)
	
	 500–1,000 mg

AMINO ACIDS (PROTEIN)	TOTAL DAILY AMOUNT
Tyrosine L-5 hydroxytryptophan (5HTP, a natural precursor of serotonin) Methionine Glutathione	200–500 mg 25–50 mg 200–500 mg 200–500 mg

*I recommend Shaklee's *Essential Omega-3 Complex*, a safe and clinically proven fish oil supplement derived from cold-water fish rich in EPA and DHA. It's easy to take in capsule form and has no odor.

†I recommend Shaklee's *GLA Plus*, which contains gamma linoleic acid, a fatty acid our bodies use to form prostaglandins—potent hormonelike substances that help the body regulate many normal bodily processes.

important phytonutrients in the right amounts. In addition, you can add Shaklee's *CoQHeart™*, which provides 30 mg of coenzyme Q_{10} in a highly bioavailable form.

It may be very difficult to find a source for the above amino acids listed on page 183. Again, don't worry; just do the best you can. If you can't find these supplements, one way to get most of these (with the exception of 5HTP) is to consume a high-quality, low-fat protein source (one that provides all the essential amino acids you need). I recommend the use of soy protein because of its full complement of essential amino acids and link to numerous health benefits. One of the best products out there is Shaklee's *Energizing Soy Protein,* which is low in fat, naturally cholesterol- and lactose-free, provides nine essential amino acids that your body needs but can't manufacture itself, and actually tastes good.

DETOXERS	TOTAL DAILY AMOUNT
*Milk thistle**	300 mg
Soluble fiber†	
Grapefruit pectin	up to 3 g before meals (three times a day)
or	
Apple pectin	up to 3 g before meals (three times a day)
or	
Psyllium seed husks	up to 3 g before meals (three times a day)

*The liver is one of our primary organs responsible for processing and eliminating contaminants and toxins. Milk thistle seed extract has been shown in research to support the body's normal ability to make proteins that help regenerate liver cells. Shaklee's *Liver DTX Complex* is an excellent milk thistle seed extract product that contains other liver detoxification ingredients and helps maintain essential bile flow.
†A good source of soluble fiber is the *Shaklee Fiber Plan®* line of products, ranging from drinks with psyllium seed husk to fiber tablets. I also recommend Shaklee's *Slim Plan Gold™* meal replacement shake, which has a full 8 grams of soluble fiber.
All soluble-fiber supplements must be taken with water as instructed. Other sources of soluble fiber are also acceptable such as other fruit pectins, and guar and acacia gums.

An important note on timing supplement doses: If you prefer, you can take all the supplements, essential fats, and protein (or amino acids) in the morning. But if you can manage it, split the dose by taking some in the morning and some in the evening. A split dose is particularly useful for vitamin C, which lasts for only about eight hours in the body. If you take the total daily amount in two doses, you will give your *Slimming System* better protection from free radicals.

One thing to remember: Whenever you take the supplements, it is important not to take them at the same time you take the detoxers, because taking the supplements and detoxers too close together increases the chance that the detoxers may "soak up" some of the essential nutrients.

Ideally, you should take the detoxers with some water as soon as you wake up in the morning, then by the time you have dressed and had breakfast you can take the supplements, leaving at least thirty minutes between the two and longer if possible.

If you want to split the vitamin doses through the day, then taking the detoxers before meals and the supplements after meals will allow sufficient time between them.

Foods to Eat Freely

Before I launch into the nitty-gritty of the diet itself, here is the good news: You can freely eat any of the following foods, provided they are organic or low in *Chemical Calories*:

- Herbs, spices, mustard, chilies, garlic, pepper, salt, soy sauce, lemon juice, vinegar, Worcestershire sauce, bouillon, fat-free vegetable soup
- Certain organic or peeled vegetables eaten raw, steamed, or as fat-free vegetable soup (see list on page 204)
- Caffeine-free coffee or tea, coffee substitutes, herbal teas, filtered water

Organic lemon or lime slices can be added freely. You can add milk, but only if it is taken from your daily allowance.

Top Tips to Ensure Success

Here are a few ideas to help you deal with temptation when the going gets tough:

- Keep some prepared raw or cooked vegetables in your refrigerator at all times for emergency snacks.
- Eat a bowl of fresh organic salad every day.
- For a hot, filling snack, have a mug of fat-free vegetable soup. You can make it in batches using the vegetables listed above and keep it in the fridge or freezer for an instant filler in emergencies. Take some with you in a Thermos when you go to work or travel.
- Drink an 8-ounce glass of filtered water before every meal and throughout the day. As well as keeping you well hydrated, drinking plenty of water will also help flush away unwanted chemicals released by your weight loss. To aid detoxification even more, drink mineral water and flavor it with lemon or lime juice.
- Remove all visible skin and fat from meat and fatty fish when preparing them for cooking.
- Don't eat the skin or fat on cooked meats.

Sometimes, though, all of us need a little extra help fighting our food cravings and resisting an unhealthy snack. Again, Shaklee has come up with three remarkable products that give you that extra help.

Shaklee's *Craving Reduction Complex* is a remarkable natural product formulated to help sustain energy and prevent rapid blood sugar declines that can lead to food cravings.

Shaklee's *Appetite Reducing Spray* is a clinically proven homeopathic spray containing sixteen ingredients to help detoxify your system and restore metabolic balance as well as relieve excessive appetite, occasional feelings of fatigue, excess water retention, occasional nervousness, and occasional indigestion.

Shaklee's *Slim Plan Gold*™ shake is a meal replacement product that provides 8 grams of soluble fiber. It also has 35 percent of the recommended daily intake of twenty-three vitamins and minerals, is 99 percent lactose-free, and is formulated to prevent blood sugar swings that can lead to food cravings or between-meal snacking.

How the Diet Is Designed

You can choose what you'd like to eat every day from six different food groups: breads/starches, lean meat (proteins), vegetables, fruit, milk, and fats/oil. You have a certain number of servings from each group, and within that number of servings you are free to make your own selection from the choices offered. Provided that you keep to the recommended portions, the nutritional value of the foods has already been counted for you, so you can relax on that front.

It is also a good idea to weigh or measure the portions at the beginning, as this will help you estimate the right quantities involved. Don't forget that you can combine your servings with as many items as you want from the "foods to eat freely" section shown above.

But whatever selections you make, you should try to keep a journal of all the food you eat as you go along. This will make it much easier to re-member how many food-group servings are still available as the day goes on and will really help you to stick to the diet.

Three Steps to Mild Food Restriction

The first step to beginning a mild food-restriction diet is choosing a food plan that works best for you. For your convenience, I have provided three different plans to choose from, with a range of calorie levels: 1,200, 1,500, and 1,800.

With the chart in Step I, choose the calorie level best designed to help you release stored *Chemical Calories* and maximize your weight loss results but one that is not so restrictive that you are constantly hungry and find it hard to stick to the diet. For men, I recommend the 1,800-calorie plan. For women, the 1,200- or 1,500-calorie plan is best; if you exercise thirty min-utes a day, consider the 1,500-calorie plan. For each calorie plan in Step I, I have listed the number of portions of each food group allowed for every meal.

Second, take a look at the sample menu plans in Step II to get ideas for meals and how to spread your servings out throughout the day. Remember that when you are choosing foods to eat, you should select those that are lowest in *Chemical Calories*. To make this task easier, I have included a chart listing various foods and where they fall in terms of being very low, low, medium, high, or very high in *Chemical Calories*.

Third, you will find below a guide to portion sizes. Use the guide to help you find foods in each food group and the appropriate serving size to build your own meals. Remember that you need to match the servings with the correct portion size to stay within the calorie range you have selected.

STEP I: CHOOSE YOUR MEAL PLAN

SERVINGS OF	1,200-CALORIE PLAN	1,500-CALORIE PLAN	1,800-CALORIE PLAN
BREAKFAST A meal replacement shake or foods listed below.*			
Lean Meat/Protein	2	2	2
Fruit	2½	2½	2½
Starch	0	0	1
Fats/Oil	0	0	1
LUNCH			
Bread/Starch	2	2	2
Lean Meat/Protein	3	3	3
Vegetable	1	2	2
Nonfat Milk	1	1	1
Fats/Oil	1	2	2
Fruit	1	1	2

*If you use a shake for your morning meal, subtract two lean meats and one and one half fruits from your daily allowances. You may want to try Shaklee's 200-calorie *Slim Plan Gold*™ shake in chocolate or vanilla flavor.

Dinner			
Bread/Starch	1	1	2
Lean Meat/Protein	3	4	4
Vegetable	1	2	2
Nonfat Milk	0	0	0
Fats/Oil	2	3	3
Fruit	0	1	1

These flexible meal plans are suggestions to help you achieve your weight loss goals. Below are example meals for four days in each of the calorie plans. If you prefer small meals and frequent snacks, you may use food from one of the meals as a between-meal snack. As an example, you could save the fruit from breakfast to eat mid-morning or the fruit from lunch to eat mid-afternoon. If, for example, you don't drink milk or use it on cereal at breakfast time, you can choose to use your milk serving at another mealtime.

STEP 2: SAMPLE MENU PLANS

Meal Ideas: 1,200 Calories*

Breakfast	Breakfast	Breakfast	Breakfast
3 tbsp. soy protein powder mixed with 8 ozs. orange juice	3 tbsp. soy protein powder mixed with 8 ozs. orange juice	3 tbsp. soy protein powder mixed with 8 ozs. orange juice	3 tbsp. soy protein powder mixed with 8 ozs. orange juice
½ cup organic blueberries	½ apple, peeled or organic	½ orange, peeled	½ cup organic raspberries

LUNCH	LUNCH	LUNCH	LUNCH
Turkey Sandwich 3 ozs. low fat turkey, 2 slices bread, 1 tbsp. low-fat mayonnaise 1 cup carrot sticks, peeled or organic 1 apple, peeled or organic 1 cup skim milk	Caesar Salad 2 ozs. chicken breast, 1 tbsp. Parmesan cheese, 1 cup organic romaine lettuce, 1 tbsp. low-fat Caesar dressing 2 slices bread 1 orange, peeled 1 cup skim milk	Hamburger 3 ozs. lean hamburger (organic, if available), 1 hamburger bun Green Salad 1 cup organic greens, 1 tbsp. nonfat dressing 1 orange, peeled 1 cup skim milk	Roast Beef Sandwich 3 ozs. low-fat roast beef, 2 slices bread, 1 tbsp. low-fat mayonnaise 1 cup carrot sticks, peeled or organic ½ banana 1 cup skim milk

DINNER	DINNER	DINNER	DINNER
Burrito 1 tortilla, 2 ozs. lean hamburger (organic, if available), 1 oz. low-fat cheese Green Salad 1 cup organic salad greens, 2 tbsp. low-fat dressing	Spaghetti ½ cup spaghetti, 2½ ozs. lean meatballs, ½ cup marinara sauce, 1 tbsp. Parmesan cheese Green Salad 1 cup organic salad greens, 1 tbsp. low-fat dressing	Chicken and Potato 3 ozs. chicken breast, ½ cup mashed potatoes ½ cup cooked organic broccoli with 2 tbsp. low-fat margarine	Beef and Potato 3 ozs. lean beef, 1 small baked potato ½ cup cooked green beans with 2 tbsp. low-fat margarine

*Measuring units: tbsp. = tablespoon, tsp. = teaspoon

Meal Ideas: 1,500 Calories*

BREAKFAST	BREAKFAST	BREAKFAST	BREAKFAST
3 tbsp. soy protein powder mixed with 8 ozs. orange juice	3 tbsp. soy protein powder mixed with 8 ozs. orange juice	3 tbsp. soy protein powder mixed with 8 ozs. orange juice	3 tbsp. soy protein powder mixed with 8 ozs. orange juice
½ cup organic blueberries	½ apple, peeled or organic	½ orange, peeled	½ cup organic raspberries

LUNCH	LUNCH	LUNCH	LUNCH
Turkey Sandwich 3 ozs. low-fat turkey, 2 slices bread, 1 tbsp. low-fat mayonnaise 1 cup carrot sticks (peeled or organic), 1 cup raw cauliflower, 1 tbsp. low-fat dressing 1 apple, peeled or organic 1 cup skim milk	Caesar Salad 2 ozs. chicken breast, 1 tbsp. Parmesan cheese, 1 cup organic romaine lettuce, 1 cup chopped tomato, 2 tbsp. low-fat Caesar dressing 2 slices bread 1 orange, peeled 1 cup skim milk	Hamburger 3 ozs. lean hamburger (organic, if available), 1 hamburger bun Salad 1 cup organic greens, 1 cup carrot sticks (peeled or organic), 2 tbsp. nonfat dressing 1 orange, peeled 1 cup skim milk	Roast Beef Sandwich 3 ozs. low-fat roast beef, 2 slices bread, 1 tbsp. low-fat mayonnaise 1 cup carrot sticks (peeled or organic), 1 cup raw organic broccoli, 1 tbsp. low-fat dressing ½ banana 1 cup skim milk

DINNER	DINNER	DINNER	DINNER
Burrito 1 tortilla, 3 ozs. lean hamburger (organic, if available), 1 oz. low-fat cheese, 1 tbsp. low-fat sour cream Salad 1 cup organic salad greens, 1 cup carrot sticks (peeled or organic), 2 tbsp. low-fat dressing ¾ cup organic blueberries	Spaghetti ½ cup spaghetti, 3½ ozs. lean meatballs, ½ cup marinara sauce, 1 tbsp. Parmesan cheese Green Salad 1 cup organic salad greens, 2 tbsp. low-fat dressing 1 apple, peeled or organic	Chicken and Potato 4 ozs. chicken breast, ½ cup mashed potatoes ½ cup cooked organic broccoli with 2 tbsp. low-fat margarine Green salad 1 cup organic salad greens, 1 tbsp. low-fat dressing ¾ cup organic blueberries	Beef and Potato 4 ozs. lean beef, 1 small baked potato ½ cup cooked green beans with 2 tbsp. low-fat margarine 1 cup carrot sticks (peeled or organic), 1 tbsp. low-fat dressing 1 cup organic raspberries

*Measuring units: tbsp. = tablespoon, tsp. = teaspoon

Meal Ideas: 1,800 Calories*

BREAKFAST	BREAKFAST	BREAKFAST	BREAKFAST
3 tbsp. soy protein powder mixed with 8 ozs. orange juice ½ cup organic blueberries 1 slice bread with 1 tsp. low-fat margarine	3 tbsp. soy protein powder mixed with 8 ozs. orange juice ½ apple, peeled or organic ½ bagel with 1 tbsp. low-fat cream cheese	3 tbsp. soy protein powder mixed with 8 ozs. orange juice ½ orange, peeled 1 slice bread with 1 tsp. low-fat margarine	3 tbsp. soy protein powder mixed with 8 ozs. orange juice ½ cup organic raspberries ½ bagel with 1 tbsp. low-fat cream cheese

LUNCH	LUNCH	LUNCH	LUNCH
Turkey Sandwich	Caesar Salad	Hamburger	Roast Beef
3 ozs. low-fat turkey, 2 slices bread, 1 tbsp. low-fat mayonnaise	2 ozs. chicken breast, 1 tbsp. Parmesan cheese, 1 cup organic romaine lettuce, 1 cup chopped tomato, 2 tbsp. low-fat Caesar dressing	3 ozs. lean hamburger (organic, if available), 1 hamburger bun	Sandwich 3 ozs. low-fat roast beef, 2 slices bread, 1 tbsp. low-fat mayonnaise
1 cup carrot sticks (peeled or organic), 1 cup raw cauliflower, 1 tbsp. low-fat dressing	2 slices bread	Green Salad 1 cup organic greens, 1 cup carrot sticks (peeled or organic), 2 tbsp. nonfat dressing	1 cup carrot sticks (peeled or organic), 1 cup raw organic broccoli, 1 tbsp. low-fat dressing
1 apple, peeled or organic	1 apple, peeled or organic	1 banana	1 banana
1 orange, peeled	1 orange, peeled	1 cup skim milk	1 cup skim milk
1 cup skim milk	1 cup skim milk		

DINNER	DINNER	DINNER	DINNER
Burrito	Spaghetti	Chicken and Potato	Beef and Potato
2 tortillas, 3 ozs. lean hamburger (organic, if available), 1 oz. low-fat cheese, 1 tbsp. low-fat sour cream	1 cup spaghetti, 3½ ozs. lean meatballs, ½ cup marinara sauce, 1 tbsp. Parmesan cheese	4 ozs. chicken breast, 1 cup mashed potatoes	4 ozs. lean beef, 1 small baked potato
Green Salad 1 cup organic salad greens, 1 cup carrot sticks (peeled or organic), 2 tbsp. low-fat dressing	Green Salad 1 cup organic salad greens, 2 tbsp. low-fat dressing	Green Salad 1 cup organic salad greens, 1 tbsp. low-fat dressing	½ cup cooked green beans 2 tbsp. low-fat margarine, 1 slice bread
¾ cup organic blueberries	1 apple, peeled or organic	½ cup cooked organic broccoli with 2 tbsp. low-fat margarine	1 cup carrot sticks (peeled or organic), 1 tbsp. low-fat dressing
		¾ cup organic blueberries	1 cup organic raspberries

*Measuring units: tbsp. = tablespoon, tsp. = teaspoon

STEP 3: GUIDE TO PORTIONS

To help you choose the right portion of food from the food groups, here is a general guide for your use.

Group 1: Breads/Starches

Depending on your calorie level, you can eat three to five servings of breads/starches every day. This works out to be three portions for those on the 1,200-calorie plan, three for those on the 1,500-calorie plan, and five for those on the 1,800-calorie plan. A typical portion of bread/starch is the following:

1 slice bread
½ bagel
½ cup dry or cooked cereal
½ cup rice or cooked pasta

Starchy vegetables, legumes, and crackers are included in this group as well. Examples of their portion size are:

½ cup corn
1 small baked potato, no skin
½ cup cooked beans
3 (2½-inch) graham crackers

Group 2: Fruit

Once again, depending on your calorie level, every day you can choose up to five and a half portions of fruit. This works out to be three and a half portions for those on the 1,200-calorie plan, four and a half for those on the 1,500-calorie plan, and five and a half for those on the 1,800-calorie plan. These are great for giving you instant energy if you need a quick pick-me-up.
A typical serving of fresh fruit is:

1 apple
1 orange
1 grapefruit

2 medium plums
1 nectarine
1 peach
1 small banana or half of a large one
¼ cup of dried fruit

Group 3: Vegetables

Depending on your calorie level, you can choose two to four servings a day from the vegetable group. This works out to be two portions for those on the 1,200-calorie plan, and four for those on the 1,500- or 1,800-calorie plans. A typical serving of vegetables is 1 cup raw vegetables or ½ cup cooked vegetables without added fat. Remember: A number of vegetables can be eaten in unlimited amounts. Those are listed on page 204.

Group 4: Lean Meat or Soy (Proteins)

Depending on your calorie level, you can choose eight to nine portions of lean meat or protein every day. This works out to be eight portions for those on the 1,200-calorie plan and nine for those on the 1,500 and 1,800-calorie plans. The following are options to choose from and their appropriate serving sizes:

1 oz. cooked lean meat (venison, beef, lamb, chicken, pork, ham, turkey)
1 oz. low-fat hard cheese or ½ oz. regular hard cheese (see guide)
¼ cup low-fat cottage cheese
1 egg (but don't eat more than 4 whole eggs per week)
2 ozs. tofu
½ cup soy protein

Group 5: Milk

You can choose one serving from the milk group every day. Because milk servings are fairly limited in the suggested meal plans, it will be important to take extra supplemental calcium and vitamin D to meet your needs for these nutrients. Refer to the list of essential supplements for recommended levels of both calcium and vitamin D.

A typical serving from the milk group is:

1 cup nonfat or 1% milk
1 cup nonfat unflavored yogurt or 1 cup reduced-calorie flavored
    yogurt
1 cup soy milk

Group 6: Fats/Oil

It's particularly important to measure out these portions of fats and keep your consumption within the quantities given. Depending on your calorie level, you can choose three to six portions from the fat/oil group every day. This works out to be three portions for those on the 1,200-calorie plan, five for those on the 1,500-calorie plan, and six for those on the 1,800-calorie plan.

1 teaspoon oil (use an oil high in monounsaturated fat, such as
    organic olive oil, for all cooking purposes and walnut oil,
    sesame oil, organic olive oil, etc., for salad dressings)
1 teaspoon organic safflower margarine (soft or liquid)
1 oz. nuts or seeds, or a combination of both (particularly walnuts)
1 tsp. nut spreads (not peanut)
1 teaspoon regular organic salad dressing or 1 tablespoon
    reduced-calorie or fat-free dressing.

You should take omega-3 and omega-6 essential oil supplements in addition to the above suggested amounts of oils/fats.

How Much Food Should You Eat?

When you first start, you will probably find that you need all the calories that are listed, and you should make the most of the foods that can be eaten freely, particularly the soup. But as the weeks go by and you approach your ideal weight, you will find it easier to eat less. Do realize that it is perfectly fine to cut back slightly on your servings if you find you don't need so much food. Just because the diet allots a certain amount of a food, that doesn't mean you have to eat it all. In other words, you should eat what you need, then stop. Pay close attention to your body's natural signs for both hunger and satiety. Eat when you first feel hungry, and don't wait too long to eat (when you are overly hungry), because then you may eat more than you actually need or make poor food choices. And remember: Stop eating when you feel comfortable, not when you necessarily feel "stuffed" or "full." Paying special attention to your hunger and satiety levels can help you naturally control the amount of food you eat.

Foods and Drinks to Avoid

There are some foods that you should definitely avoid on the *Chemical Calorie* Detox Diet, because they slow down or impair your ability to detoxify. They include:

- Caffeinated drinks, because they disturb the production of slimming hormones and create carbohydrate cravings (see Chapter 16).
- Alcohol, because it slows down detoxification. For this reason, it is particularly important for you to avoid it in the first week of food restriction (see Chapter 16).
- Diet sodas, because they are high-acidity drinks
- Foods high in trans-fats. Trans-fats are created when even good fat, such as polyunsaturated oil, is heated in cooking. For example, sunflower oil is a healthy oil unless it is heated to high temperatures, such as when frying foods and thereby creating trans-fats. Limit yourself to cooking with olive oil from your allowed number of servings. Many kinds of margarines are also high in trans-fats, so look for brands of margarines that are free of them.
- Foods very high in *Chemical Calories* (see *Chemical Calorie* Food List in this chapter).

The *Chemical Calorie* Food Guide

These *Chemical Calorie* food charts are what losing weight is all about. With this new and totally revolutionary guide to the typical *Chemical Calorie* levels in foods, you will be able for the first time ever to get a good idea of which foods are likely to make you fat and which are not, and in the process you may see many of your favorite foods in a completely new light.

HOW THESE CHARTS WERE PRODUCED

To produce these charts, I have used four sets of nationally published and publicly available data from the U.S. Food and Drug Administration (FDA) Total Diet Study, an ongoing food-testing program that regularly monitors pesticide residues in food.[4] Using data from more than ninety different kinds of pesticides, I calculated the average number of *Chemical Calories* for each food. As all the foods were tested four times, I then worked out the average number of *Chemical Calories* for each particular food.

HOW TO USE THE CHARTS

In order to keep things simple, I have created five categories that will indicate the level of *Chemical Calories* found in each food. These categories are as follows:

- Very low
- Low
- Medium
- High
- Very high

A brief summary of each of these categories, as follows, will enable you to use them best.

The foods in the *very low* category are the safest, as they either have no measurable or extremely low levels of *Chemical Calories* detected. Of course, these foods should still be washed thoroughly before eating.

The foods in the *low* category are still relatively safe, as the average level detected in these foods remains reasonably low. But still wash or peel fruits or vegetables thoroughly just to be on the safe side.

When you look at the foods with *medium* levels of chemicals, you can see that it becomes more worthwhile to consider buying an organic version if available, as these foods can contain significant levels of *Chemical Calories*. If no organic alternative is available, you can use the techniques described in Chapter 9 to lower any potential contamination.

With foods found to have *high* levels of *Chemical Calories*, the problem becomes much more serious, as these levels, over time, could significantly damage your *Slimming System*. So stepping up your efforts to avoid these foods will be definitely worth your while. Again, do look for an organic option or use appropriate methods of preparation to lower potential contamination.

Finally, the foods in the *very high* category should be avoided if possible and the organic alternative substituted wherever appropriate.

EXPLAINING THE VARIABILITY OF DIFFERENT FOODS

One thing to bear in mind is that these levels are based on the average levels of *pesticides* found in the relatively small samples of foods tested by the FDA. This means that the amounts of *Chemical Calories* will be totally dependent on the farming practices used for those particular foods. As practices can vary greatly, the guide can provide only a rough estimate of how contaminated the foods you choose to eat might be.

And as you go through the different categories, you will find that some foods may be high in *Chemical Calories* in one form but lower in another. This may be because processing often lowers the level of pesticides in the food as certain *Chemical Calories* are broken down by heat. But despite the tendency of processed foods to be lower in *Chemical Calories,* you should not eat more processed foods at the expense of foods with higher levels of nutrients, such as fruits and vegetables.

The simple act of preparing fruits and vegetable for the table appears to play an important role in determining how many *Chemical Calories* you will have in your meals. All the foods in the food chart have been tested after they have been prepared, and you can clearly see the positive effect of removing the skin. You will notice that unpeeled baked white potatoes contain much higher levels of *Chemical Calories* than the peeled and boiled white potatoes. So by all means make washing and peeling your fruits and vegetables a must whenever possible. When it comes to such foods as lettuce, broccoli, and green peppers, it is probably best to buy organic if you can. Interestingly, cauliflower, probably because it has outer leaves to protect it from chemicals, is lower in *Chemical Calories* than other vegetables. In contrast, broccoli is not so protected, so if the chemical cannot be removed by washing, it will remain on the food.

However, you can also see that in some cases even peeling does not appear to reduce the *Chemical Calorie* load of a food. This could be because the kinds of pesticides used on it work systemically. In other words, they work by penetrating the body of the fruit rather than just by sitting on the surface. The *Chemical Calorie* charts reflect all these differences.

I also need to mention meat, dairy, and eggs here. As these charts have been based on the level of pesticides detected in foods, much of this produce appears to be relatively low in *Chemical Calories*. However, this produce can also contain antibiotics, other growth promoters, and environmental pollutants, which were not tested for these FDA reports. As many of these chemicals can also possess weight promotion abilities, they will also potentially contain a certain amount of *Chemical Calories*. This could be the case in the meat and products of intensively farmed animals, such as chickens, turkeys, and pigs, actually being much higher in *Chemical Calories* than these initial charts first suggest. To deal with this possibility, I will be reevaluating all animals and animal produce for these additional added chemicals, and although these results cannot be provided in this book because of time restraints, when they become available they will appear on my website, www.slimmingsystems.com, as well as in future publications.

Last of all, remember that these levels are not cast in stone and will need to be continually updated. Because the chemicals used on crops keep changing, these charts will need to be renewed every few years to keep up with the changes in agriculture. So as the years go by, you should expect the overall level of *Chemical Calories* for different foods to change. I will make sure that those changes are reflected on our website.

The Food List

The food list includes foods in each of the groups in the food plan. You can use any food in a food group to satisfy a "serving" of that group. Do not exchange food groups; your calorie count will not remain within your food group. For example, if you tried to exchange one vegetable serving (typically 40 to 50 calories) for one milk serving (80 calories), you would be consuming almost double the number of calories that you intended.

Always look at the serving size on the food list. Calorie-dense foods (nuts, meats) have small serving sizes, and foods with fewer calories (raw vegetables) have much larger serving sizes. There are some "free foods"— foods that you may consume without counting the servings.

MEASUREMENT OF FOODS

It is important to eat the right serving sizes of food. You will need to learn how to estimate the amount of food you are served. You can do this by measuring all the food you eat for a week or so. Measure liquids with a measuring cup. Some solid foods (such as tuna, cottage cheese, and canned fruits) can also be measured with a measuring cup. Use measuring spoons for smaller amounts of other foods (such as oil, salad dressing, and peanut butter). A scale can be very useful for measuring almost anything, especially meat, poultry, and fish. All food should be measured or weighed after cooking.

Some food that you buy uncooked will weigh less after you cook it. This is true of most meats. Starches often swell during cooking, so a small amount of uncooked starch will become a much larger amount of cooked food. The following table shows some of the changes:

Starch Group	Uncooked	Cooked	*Chemical Calorie* Level
Oatmeal	3 level tbsp.	½ cup	Very low
Cream of wheat	2 level tbsp.	½ cup	Very low
Grits	3 level tbsp.	½ cup	Very low
Rice, white	2 level tbsp.	⅓ cup	Low
Spaghetti	¼ cup	½ cup	Very low
Noodles	⅓ cup	½ cup	Very low
Macaroni	¼ cup	½ cup	Very low
Dried beans	3 tbsp.	⅓ cup	Very low
Dried peas	3 tbsp.	⅓ cup	Very low
Lentils	2 tbsp.	⅓ cup	Very low
Meat group			
Hamburger	4 ozs.	3 ozs.	High
Chicken	½ whole chicken breast	3 ozs.	Very low

FREE FOODS

A free food is any food or drink that contains fewer than twenty calories per serving. You can eat as much as you want of items that have no serving size specified. You may eat two or three servings per day of those items that have a specific serving size listed. Be sure to spread them out through the day.

Drinks	*Chemical Calorie* Level
Water, filtered	Very low
Carbonated water	Very low
Coffee, decaffeinated	Very low
Lemon juice	Very low

Lime juice	Very low
Tea, decaffeinated	Very low

VEGETABLES, RAW (1 CUP)

Bean sprouts, boiled	Very low
Cabbage, fresh, boiled	Very low
Carrots (organic)	Very low
Celery	High
Celery (organic)	Very low
Cucumber	High
Cucumber (organic)	Very low
Green onion	Medium
Jalapeño peppers, fresh	Medium
Mushrooms	Medium
Radishes	High
Radishes (organic)	Very low
Zucchini	Very high
Zucchini (organic)	Very low
Salad greens (organic)	Very low
Endive (organic)	Very low
Iceberg lettuce	Medium
Iceberg lettuce (organic)	Very low
Romaine lettuce (organic)	Very low
Escarole (organic)	Very low

CONDIMENTS

Catsup (1 tbsp.)	Low
Chilis, dried	Low
Chili powder	Low
Mustard	Medium
Soy sauce, regular or lite	Very low
Vinegar	Very low
Nonstick pan spray, using the minimum amount	Low

STARCH/BREAD LIST

You can choose your starch servings from any of the items on this list. If you want to eat a starch food that is not on the list, the general rule is this:

½ cup cereal, grain, or pasta = one serving
1 ounce of a bread product = one serving

CEREALS/GRAINS/PASTA		CHEMICAL CALORIE LEVEL
Bran cereals, concentrated (such as Bran Buds, All Bran)	⅓ cup	Low
Bran cereals, flaked	½ cup	Low
Bran cereals with raisins	½ cup	Medium
Bulgur (cooked)	½ cup	Medium
Oatmeal, quick (cooked)	½ cup	Very low
Farina, wheat (cooked)	½ cup	Very low
Cornmeal, dry	2½ tbsp.	Very low
Grits (cooked)	½ cup	Very low
Cereal, corn flakes	½ cup	Very low
Cereal, oat rings	½ cup	Very low
Cereal, crisped rice	½ cup	Very low
Cereal, shredded wheat	½ cup	Very low
Pasta, macaroni	½ cup	Very low
Pasta, noodle	½ cup	Very low
Pasta, spaghetti	½ cup	Very low
Pasta, rice noodles	½ cup	Very low
Rice, white or brown (cooked)	⅓ cup	Very low
DRIED BEANS/PEAS/LENTILS		
Beans, black, dried (cooked)	⅓ cup	Very low
Beans, kidney, dried (cooked)	⅓ cup	Very low

Beans, pinto, dried (cooked)	⅓ cup	Very low
Lentils (cooked)	⅓ cup	Very low
Peas, dried (cooked)	⅓ cup	Very low
Baked beans	¼ cup	Very low

STARCHY VEGETABLES

Corn, fresh/frozen (boiled)	½ cup	Very low
Corn on the cob, fresh/frozen (boiled)	6-inch cob	Very low
Lima beans, fresh/frozen (boiled)	½ cup	Medium
Peas, green, canned or frozen	½ cup	Medium
Potato, baked, with skin	3 ozs.	High
Potato, no skin (baked or boiled)	3 ozs.	Low
Potato, mashed	½ cup	Low
Squash, winter (acorn, butternut) fresh/frozen (boiled)	¾ cup	High
Yam, sweet potato	⅓ cup	Very low

BREAD

Bagel, ½	(1 oz.)	Low
English muffin	½	Very low
Frankfurter or hamburger bun	½ (1 oz.)	Low
Pita, 6 in. across	½	Low
Plain roll, small	1 (1 oz.)	Low
Rye, pumpernickel	1 slice (1 oz.)	Low
Tortilla, corn, 6 in. across	1	Low
Tortilla, wheat, 6 in. across	1	Low
White (including French, Italian)	1 slice (1 oz.)	Medium
Whole wheat	1 slice	Medium

CRACKERS/SNACKS

Graham crackers, 2½ in. square	3	Low
Matzoh	¾ oz.	Low
Melba toast	5 slices	Low
Oyster crackers	24	Low
Popcorn, no fat added (popped)	3 cups	Low
Pretzels	¾ oz.	Low
Rye crisp (2 in. × 3½ in.)	4	Very low
Saltine-type crackers	6	Low
Whole-wheat crackers, no fat added (crisp breads such as Finn, Kavli, Wasa)	2–4 slices (¾ oz.)	Low

STARCHY FOODS PREPARED WITH FAT

(count as 1 starch/bread serving, plus 1 fat serving)

Biscuit, 2½ in. across	1	Very low
Chow mein noodles	½ cup	Medium
Corn bread, 2-in. cube	1 (2 ozs.)	Very low
Cracker, round butter type	6	Very low
Chips, corn, 1 oz. = 1 bread, 2 fat	12	Low
French-fried potatoes (2 in. to 3½ in. long)	10 (1½ oz.)	Medium
Muffin, plain, small	1	Very low
Pancake, 4 in. across	2	Low
Taco shell	2 (6 in. across)	Medium
Waffle	1 (4½ in. square)	Medium
Whole-wheat crackers, fat added (such as Triscuits)	4–6 (1 oz.)	Low

LEAN MEAT AND SUBSTITUTES

Some commonly consumed portions of meat, soy, and cheese are:

- Chicken breast: skinless, 3 ounces equals three meat servings
- Lean beef: 3 ounces (size of a deck of cards) equals three meat servings
- Lean hamburger: 3 oz (size of a deck of cards) equals three meat servings
- Regular cheese (100 or more calories per ounce): 1 ounce equals two meat servings
- Soy protein: ½ cup equals 3.5 meat servings

Lean Meat and Substitutes		
ONE SERVING IS EQUAL TO ANY ONE OF THE FOLLOWING ITEMS:		*CHEMICAL CALORIES*
BEEF		
USDA Good or Choice grades of lean beef, such as round, sirloin, and flank steak; tenderloin	1 oz.	Medium
Lean Hamburger	1 oz.	High
95% fat-free beef lunch meat	1 oz.	Medium
95% fat-free pastrami lunch meat	1 oz.	Medium
95% fat-free bologna lunch meat	1 oz.	Medium

PORK		
Chop	1 oz.	Very low
Bacon, turkey, 1 oz. = 1 meat + 1 fat	2 slices	Medium
Sausage, low-fat, 1 link = 1 meat	1 link	Medium
Ham	1 oz.	Very low
Roast	1 oz.	Very low
Sausage	1 oz.	Medium
95% fat-free ham lunch meat	1 oz.	Very low

POULTRY		
Chicken, breast (without skin)	1 oz.	Very low
Turkey breast (without skin)	1 oz.	Very low
95% fat-free turkey lunch meat	1 oz.	Very low

FISH		
Salmon	1 oz.	Very high
Halibut	1 oz.	Low
Fish sticks	1 oz.	Very low
Crab	2 ozs.	Low
Shrimp (boiled)	2 ozs.	Very low
Tuna, canned in water	¼ cup	Very low
Tuna steaks, fresh or frozen	1 oz.	High
Sardines, canned	2 medium	Very low

CHEESE		
Any cottage cheese	¼ cup	Low
Grated Parmesan	2 tbsp.	Medium
Diet cheese (with fewer than 55 calories per ounce)	1 oz.	Low
Low-fat cream cheese	1 oz.	Medium

Regular American processed cheese	½ oz.	Very high
Regular Cheddar	½ oz.	High
Regular Swiss	½ oz.	High

OTHER

Egg whites	2	Very low
Eggs, whole = 1 protein + 1 fat	1	Low

SOY

Tofu and other soy products	½ cup	Very low
Soy protein drink (powdered)	2 ozs.	Very low

VEGETABLE LIST

Unless otherwise noted, the serving size for vegetables (one vegetable serving) is:

½ cup cooked vegetables or vegetable juice
1 cup raw vegetables

Note: You may increase the portion size of the non-starchy vegetables mentioned below. Starchy vegetables such as corn, peas, and potatoes are found on the Starch/Bread List. For "free" vegetables see the Free Food List.

Vegetables	Serving Size	Chemical Calories
Artichoke	(½ medium)	Medium
Asparagus, fresh or frozen	½ cup cooked 1 cup raw	Medium
Beans, green, fresh or frozen	½ cup cooked 1 cup raw	Low
Bean sprouts	½ cup cooked 1 cup raw	Very low
Beets, fresh or frozen	½ cup cooked 1 cup raw	Low
Broccoli, fresh or frozen	½ cup cooked 1 cup raw	Medium
Brussels sprouts, fresh or frozen	½ cup cooked 1 cup raw	Very low
Cauliflower, fresh or frozen	½ cup cooked 1 cup raw	Very low
Eggplant, fresh (boiled)	½ cup cooked 1 cup raw	Very low
Greens, collard	½ cup cooked 1 cup raw	Very high
Leeks	½ cup cooked 1 cup raw	Very low
Mushrooms	½ cup cooked 1 cup raw	Medium
Okra, fresh or frozen	½ cup cooked 1 cup raw	Very low
Onions	½ cup cooked 1 cup raw	Very low
Pea pods	½ cup cooked 1 cup raw	Medium
Peppers fresh, green	½ cup cooked 1 cup raw	High
Pumpkin, canned, sugar-free	1 cup	High

Sauerkraut, canned	½ cup	Very low
Spinach, fresh or frozen (cooked)	½ cup cooked	Very high
	1 cup raw	
Squash, summer (crookneck)	½ cup cooked	Very high
	1 cup raw	
Squash, summer (crookneck), organic	½ cup cooked	Very low
	1 cup raw	
Tomato (1 large)	1 large	Low
Tomato/vegetable juice	½ cup	Very low
Tomato sauce (pasta)	½ cup	Low
Water chestnut	½ cup cooked	Very low

FRUIT LIST

Use fresh fruits or frozen or canned fruits with no sugar added. Whole fruit is more filling than fruit juice and may be a better choice for those who are trying to lose weight. Unless otherwise noted, the size of one fruit serving is:

½ cup fresh fruit or fruit juice
¼ cup dried fruit

FRESH, FROZEN, AND UNSWEETENED CANNED FRUIT		CHEMICAL CALORIES
Apples, raw (2 in. across)	1	Very high
Apples peeled, raw (2 in. across)	1	Low
Apples, organic, raw (2 in. across)	1	Very low
Applesauce (unsweetened)	½ cup	Low
Apricots, canned (4 halves)	½ cup	Low
Apricots, fresh	2 medium	Low
Banana (9 in. long)	½	Low
Blackberries, raw	¾ cup	Low

Blueberries, raw	¾ cup	Medium
Cantaloupe (5 in. across)	⅓	Medium
Cantaloupe (cubes)	1 cup	Medium
Cherries, large, raw	12 whole	High
Cherries (organic)	12 whole	Low
Cranberries, fresh or frozen	1⅓ cup	Very low
Figs, raw (2 in. across)	2	Very low
Grapefruit (medium)	½	Medium
Grapes (small)	15	Medium
Honeydew melon (medium)	⅛	Very low
Honeydew melon (cubes)	1 cup	Very low
Kiwi (large)	1	Medium
Lemon, including skin	1	High
Lemon, juice only	1	Low
Lime, juice only	1	Low
Mandarin oranges	¾ cup	Low
Mango (small)	½	Very low
Nectarines (2½ in. across)	1	Medium
Orange (2½ in. across)	1	Low
Papaya	1 cup	Low
Peach (2¾ in. across)	1	High
Peaches, canned (2 halves)	1 cup	Very low
Peach, peeled (2¾ in. across)	1	Low
Peach, organic (2¾ in. across)	1	Very low
Pear (½ large)	1 small	Medium
Pears, canned (2 halves)	½ cup	Very low
Pineapple, fresh	¾ cup	Low
Pineapple, canned	⅓ cup	Very low
Plum, raw (2 in. across)	2	High
Raspberries, raw	1 cup	Medium
Strawberries, raw, whole	1¼ cup	Very high
Strawberries, raw, whole (organic)	1¼ cup	Very low
Tangerine (2½ in. across)	2	Low
Watermelon, cubes	1¼ cup	Very low

Dried Fruit

Apricots	7 halves	Very low
Dates (medium)	2½	Very low
Figs	1½	Very low
Prunes (medium)	3	Low
Raisins	2 tbsp.	Very high
Raisins (organic)	2 tbsp.	Very low

Fruit Juice

Apple juice/cider	½ cup	Low
Cranberry juice cocktail	⅓ cup	Very low
Grapefruit juice	½ cup	Very low
Grape juice	⅓ cup	Very low
Orange juice	½ cup	Very low
Pineapple juice	½ cup	Very low
Prune juice	⅓ cup	Very low

Jelly, Jam, and Sweeteners

Jelly	1 tbsp.	Very low
Jam	1 tbsp.	Low
Marmalade	1 tbsp.	Low
Sugar	1 tbsp.	Very low
Honey	1 tbsp.	Very low

MILK LIST

SKIM AND VERY-LOW-FAT MILK		CHEMICAL CALORIES
Skim milk	1 cup	Very low
2% milk	1 cup	Low
Low-fat buttermilk	1 cup	Low
Evaporated skim milk	½ cup	High
Plain nonfat yogurt	8 ozs.	Low
MILK/SOY MILK PRODUCTS		
Plain low-fat yogurt (with added nonfat milk solids)	8 ozs.	Low
Soy milk, low-fat	1 cup	Very low

FAT LIST

Each serving on the fat list contains about five grams of fat and forty-five calories. The foods on the fat list contain mostly fat, although some items may also contain a small amount of protein. All fats are high in calories and should be carefully measured. While it is essentially impossible to avoid eating any saturated fat, everyone should modify their fat intake by limiting saturated fat to less than 10 percent of their diet and substituting healthy fat for saturated fat. When shopping, look for healthy products made with less than 10 percent saturated fat.

FATS		CHEMICAL CALORIES
Avocado	⅛ medium	Very low
Butter	1 tbsp.	Very high

Low-fat cream cheese	1 tbsp.	Medium
Margarine	1 tsp.	Medium
Margarine, diet	1 tbsp.	Low
Mayonnaise	1 tsp.	Low
Mayonnaise, reduced-calorie	1 tbsp.	Very low
Salad dressing, low-fat Caesar	1 tbsp.	Very low
Salad dressing, low-fat Ranch	1 tbsp.	Very low
Salad dressing, low-fat French	2 tbsp.	Very low
Salad dressing, low-fat Italian	2 tbsp.	Very low
Sour cream	1 tsp.	High
Sour cream, low-fat	1 tbsp.	Medium

OILS

Olive	1 tsp.	High
Olive (organic)	1 tsp.	Very low
Safflower	1 tsp.	High
Safflower (organic)	1 tsp.	Very low
Canola	1 tsp.	Medium
Corn	1 tsp.	Medium
Peanut	1 tsp.	High
Soybean	1 tsp.	Low

NUTS AND SEEDS

Almonds	6	Very low
Cashews	1 tbsp.	Very low
Coconut, unsweetened	1 tsp.	Very low
Pecans	2	Very low
Peanuts, dry-roasted	15	High
Peanut butter, natural or regular	See combination foods	
Walnuts	2 whole	Very low
Mixed nuts, without peanuts	1 tbsp.	Low
Sesame seeds	1 tbsp.	Low
Olives, black or green (small)	10	Medium
Olives, black or green (large)	5	Medium

HERBS AND SPICES

Basil	Very low
Basil (organic)	Very low
Bay leaves	Medium
Chilies	Low
Chives	Low
Cinnamon	Very low
Coriander	Medium
Coriander seed	Very low
Cumin, ground	Very low
Dill	Very high
Fennel	Very low
Garlic	Very low
Garlic, chopped, dried	Very low
Ginger	Very low
Mace, ground	Very low
Marjoram	Very low
Mint	Very high
Mixed herbs	Very low
Mustard seeds	Very low
Nutmeg	Very low
Oregano	Very low
Paprika	Very low
Parsley	Medium
Parsley root	Very low
Pepper, black	Very low
Pepper, cayenne	Very low
Rosemary	Medium
Sage	Very low
Tarragon	Low
Thyme	Very low
Turmeric	Very low

COMBINATION FOODS

Much of the food we eat is mixed together in various combinations. These combination foods do not fit into only one exchange list. It can be quite hard to tell what is in a certain casserole dish or baked food item. The following is a list of average values for some typical combination foods, which will help you fit these foods into your meal plan.

Food	Amount	Exchanges	Chemical Calories
Peanut Butter (regular)	1 tbsp.	1 lean meat, 3 fats	High
Peanut Butter (organic)	1 tbsp.	1 lean meat, 3 fats	Very low
Peanut Butter, reduced-fat (organic)	1 tbsp.	1 lean meat, 2 fats	Very low
Cheese pizza, thin crust	¼ (15-oz. size) pizza or 1 (10-in.) pizza	1 medium-fat meat, 2 starches, 1 fat	High
Chili with beans (commercial)	1 cup (8 ozs.)	2 medium-fat meat, 2 starches, 2 fats	Low
Chow mein (without noodles or rice)	2 cups (16 ozs.)	2 lean meat, 1 starch, 2 vegetables	Very low
Spaghetti with tomato sauce (canned)	1 cup (8 ozs.)	1 medium-fat meat, 1 fat, 2 starches	Very low
Macaroni and cheese	1 cup (8 ozs.)	1 medium-fat meat, 2 starches, 2 fats	Low

Soup			
Bean	1 cup (8 ozs.)	1 lean meat, 1 starch, 1 vegetable	Very low
Chunky, all varieties	10¾-oz. can	1 medium-fat meat, 1 starch, 1 vegetable	Low

16

Typical Questions
and Useful Answers

For all of you who are on, or about to go on, the Body Restoration Plan Diet, this chapter contains a wealth of important and useful information. Don't skip over it, as it could really help you benefit more fully from the program.

I think by now you will have realized that I like to work on the principle that it is far better to be well informed than to be kept in the dark. Consequently, the more you understand a diet, the more you will benefit from it. Although many of your questions will have been answered in the earlier chapters, the answers here will cover a whole range of different issues to help you achieve and maintain your desired weight.

Q. *Do I need to do everything recommended in this book to lose weight?*

A. No! Adopting just a few of the recommendations will help. Since the vast majority of the most persistent *Chemical Calories* in our bodies come from our food and drink, you can make a huge difference just by buying and eating foods that are low in *Chemical Calories* and taking the appropriate dietary supplements. These are probably the two most important things you can do. If you can adopt any of the other measures recommended, that will be an additional benefit.

Q. *I can't afford to buy organic foods, so will this diet still work for me?*

A. Absolutely! If you buy and eat food that is low in *Chemical Calories* and take the required supplements, you should still be able to lose weight permanently.

Q. *I am a confirmed coffee and tea addict and wonder why they are not recommended on the diet?*

A. Caffeinated coffee and tea interfere with the Body Restoration Plan Diet in two major ways. First, they are nutrient grabbers, so they hijack many of the vitamins and minerals that your *Slimming System* needs to function properly.[1] Second, they contain caffeine, which interferes with and temporarily increases the levels of those powerful fat-burning hormones, catecholamines, in the blood, giving you that extra energy buzz. However, you will pay dearly for this boost, as caffeine also increases the rate at which these slimming hormones are dispelled from the body. So a few hours later, the levels of these hormones can slump to lower-than-normal body levels, making you feel washed out. In addition, the fall in catecholamines may encourage increased food cravings, so you may also end up eating more.[2] If you feel you cannot stop drinking coffee or tea all at once, I recommend beginning by switching to the decaffeinated varieties.

Q. *I am a heavy smoker and am afraid to quit smoking in case I put on more weight. What should I do?*

A. You are not alone. Many people are afraid to quit smoking because they think they will gain weight. When you inhale nicotine, it artificially alters the levels of certain slimming hormones, so on one level it helps control your weight in the short term. What you may not realize, though, is that many of the chemicals you inhale in cigarette smoke are very high in *Chemical Calories,* which damage your *Slimming System* in the long term.[3]

Quitting smoking may cause a temporary weight gain, but as you rid yourself of *Chemical Calories*, you will be able to regain control over your natural *Slimming System*. Don't worry, the Body Restoration Plan Diet will help you lose any initial weight gained, and in the long term it will be one of the major factors helping you get down to your desired weight.

Q. We are always being told that a certain amount of alcohol is beneficial to health, so why do we have to limit our intake of alcohol on the diet?

A. Normally, drinking moderate amounts of alcohol is not really a problem, but the situation changes when you embark on a diet. As well as guzzling up slimming nutrients, alcohol also reduces our ability to rid our bodies of *Chemical Calories*. The whole point of the Body Restoration Plan Diet is to mobilize *Chemical Calories* and get rid of them, so it would be counterproductive to slow down the process by drinking alcohol while trying to detoxify.

I do understand that for some people cutting out alcohol for the total period of the diet itself will be very difficult. If this is the case, I recommend that you try not to consume any alcohol for at least the first week, as this is the time the detox system will be under the greatest pressure. While you are restricting your food intake, you should limit your consumption to at the very most four drinks a week for women and eight for men. One drink means a single measure of spirit, a glass of wine, a small glass of sherry, or a pint of beer or lager. When you are not actively restricting calories, you can increase your intake as long as you follow nationally recommended guidelines and take your vitamin and mineral supplements. The additional vitamins (particularly the B vitamins) should boost your ability to detoxify alcohol.

Q. Can I use food that I've not eaten one day in the next day's menu?

A. I'm afraid it doesn't work like that. Any savings that you make in your food servings for one day can't be rolled over to the next day.

Q. What if I pig out and break the diet completely?

A. Don't give up! Most people will have an occasional splurge. While it is not ideal, breaking your diet from time to time is a common fact of life. As long as you limit the damage, it will just slow your weight loss. However, the more *Chemical Calories* you shed, the less you will feel the urge to break the diet.

Finding it hard to stick to the diet is often a sign that your body has very high levels of *Chemical Calories* and is deficient in many essential nutrients. So the best thing to do is stop actively reducing your food intake for a while and concentrate on cutting down on *Chemical Calories* and taking the right supplements. After a few weeks, your body may be better prepared to restart the diet, and you will be one step closer to permanent weight loss.

Q. According to your book, many of the persistent Chemical Calories *tend to be found in animal products, so will becoming a vegan help me maintain my weight?*

A. While it is generally a very good idea to eat more soy, fruit, vegetables, beans, nuts, and grains, it is not necessary to cut out meat or dairy products totally, as many of them can be low in *Chemical Calories.*

Q. How long will it take to remove all the Chemical Calories *from my body?*

A. Different chemicals are removed from the body at different rates. It is virtually impossible to remove them all, but as long as you follow the program and keep current exposure low, many chemicals can be drastically reduced in weeks. Others will take months or even longer to eliminate. On average, if you follow the program you should considerably lower your stored levels of *Chemical Calories* within a few months. When you remember that it has taken you a lifetime to build up the levels of many chemicals, clearing the majority in a few months starts to sound so much more reasonable!

Q. *How are we being damaged by these chemicals, as the actual levels in our bodies are in fact relatively low?*

A. Well, there is a very good explanation. Despite being present at relatively small levels, they bring about many of their toxic effects by damaging our hormones, which are present in even smaller amounts. These hormones are vital in orchestrating all the reactions taking place in the body.

    The consequence of lifelong exposure to these chemicals is that the average person is already polluted with chemicals at levels millions of times higher than our natural hormone levels.[4] Although synthetic chemicals tend to be far less potent than our natural hormones, their presence is very real and can cause real damage.

Q. *Don't we build up a resistance to these toxic chemicals over time?*

A. This is a commonly held belief among many people and needs to be put to rest once and for all. Chemicals are very different from bugs such as viruses and bacteria, against which our immune system has developed the ability to fight over many hundreds of thousands of years. Continually exposing our bodies to these chemicals does not build up our resistance to them. Rather, they actually seem to target and cripple the immune system itself. Consequently, the hard reality is that the more chemicals you are exposed to over time, the more damaged your immune system will tend to become, making you not only increasingly susceptible to a whole range of infections but also more prone to a large number of immune-related diseases such as allergies, eczema, asthma, and autoimmune diseases.

Q. *I have just moved into a new house that could be full of* Chemical Calories, *but how am I to find out?*

A. Calling in an environmental house doctor or leasing equipment to take air and water samples will help you identify potential problems. The previous owners may be able to tell you whether the house has been treated for wet rot, dry rot, or timber infestation, or the guarantees for these treatments may be with the house deeds. You may also be able to find out whether the previous occupants used natural cleaning and building products or standard commercial products containing chemicals.

Q. *After I went on the program, I found that my eczema greatly improved. Is this a coincidence or a side effect of the diet?*

A. Cutting out *Chemical Calories* can greatly improve eczema. Toxic chemicals are thought to be at the heart of many autoimmune disorders, so if you lower their levels and feed the body the nutrients that it needs to repair itself, you will benefit from stronger, healthier skin. You may also see improvement in other skin disorders, such as acne and dry, itchy skin.

Q. *You say that your program will help people lose weight. I don't need to lose much weight, but I would like to improve my body shape. Will it still help me?*

A. Without a doubt. In fact, this is one of the major strengths of this program. As the *Chemical Calories* are removed from the body, the hormones in charge of shaping your body as nature intended will spring into action. As a result, men will find that their muscles increase in size and they lose fat around their middles. Women will tend to lose fat from the waist, hips, and thighs, and their muscle tone will also improve.

Q. *Even when I lose weight, I still have cellulite on my thighs and hips. Will your program reduce cellulite too?*

A. Absolutely. Cellulite is the "orange-peel" dimpling that we get on our skin, particularly around the thighs, stomach, and arms. Reducing our levels of *Chemical Calories* will reduce the size of the fat cells that stretch the skin to cause the dimpling effect. In addition, our skin will become stronger and thicker due to increased production of protein-rich tissues. As a result, the dimples will become less noticeable and start to vanish.

Q. *How can I protect my* Slimming System *if I have to fast for religious purposes?*

A. The sudden release of *Chemical Calories* into the bloodstream during fasting may actually damage the *Slimming System* and the rest of the body. To minimize any damage, you need to take the supplements recommended for the diet for a few days before and after the day of the fast. In addition, you should take fiber supplements or foods rich in soluble fiber immediately before fasting and for one or two days afterward. If possible, you should also drink lots of water while you fast and reduce your level of activity.

Q. *What can I do if I am invited out to dinner and am given foods that I know are very high in* Chemical Calories?
A. This can be tricky but is not an insurmountable problem. When your hosts have gone to great trouble to prepare food, it can be rude to refuse it. The easy thing to do is to eat more of the foods that are lower in *Chemical Calories* and less of the rest. If this is not possible, you could eat the food, then when you get back home, take an extra dose of fiber and possibly some of the other binding substances mentioned in Chapter 14.

It will take you six to eight hours to fully digest your food, so the binding substances will still reduce your intake of *Chemical Calories* very significantly. Better still, you could take the binding substances just before you go out.

Q. *I adore eating salmon and can't imagine giving it up. Is there any way to buy or prepare salmon that is low in* Chemical Calories?
A. I'm afraid that will be difficult, as most salmon contains very high levels of *Chemical Calories*. Your best alternative is to choose organic salmon. Organically raised salmon lacks a whole number of chemicals that are added to ordinary farmed salmon, although it may still contain significant amounts of *Chemical Calories* from the fish's diet.

There is, however, the possibility that in the future more vegetable sources of proteins may be used to feed fish, which has the potential to significantly cut down on the overall level of *Chemical Calories*. Otherwise, the best option is to cut off all visible fat while preparing salmon, and to eat the salmon along with foods high in soluble fiber, such as peas, lentils, or beans, since they will significantly reduce your uptake of *Chemical Calories* from the fish.

Q. *My job requires me to eat out at a lot of places that do not serve organic food. How can I avoid eating too many* Chemical Calories?

A. The good thing about eating out is that you have a choice of foods. Try to order food containing lower levels of *Chemical Calories*. Better still, order dishes that are high in soluble fiber, such as peas, lentils, or beans. If you are in any doubt, you could always take a fiber supplement either before or after your meal.

Q. *I am pregnant, but I'm putting on far too much weight. My doctor says I should try to control my weight, but I am finding it almost impossible. What can I do?*

A. The first thing to emphasize is that you should fully discuss your weight management and potential supplementation program with your physician before embarking on any changes. Second, at no stage of your pregnancy should you actively restrict what you eat. This could harm your unborn baby by mobilizing your stored levels of *Chemical Calories* and could increase the baby's risk for a whole range of illnesses. However, there are many ways to prevent excessive weight gain while still protecting the health of your baby.

The most obvious thing to do is buy and eat food that is low in *Chemical Calories*. Next, you can take vitamin and mineral supplements specially designed for pregnancy, which you should check out with your physician. It is usually an excellent idea to take omega-3 supplements in the form of organic flax oil or pesticide-free fish oil, as this will help your baby's development and boost your own *Slimming System*. These measures, in combination with a diet naturally high in soluble fiber, should help you control your weight.

More and more women are now going on detoxification programs before they become pregnant. The full program contained in this book would be ideal for any woman who is considering becoming pregnant in the future but who is not yet actively trying.

Q. Despite my best efforts, my five-year-old son seems to be putting on too much weight. What can I do to help him?

A. More and more children are becoming overweight, but the good news is that there are lots of things you can do to reverse the trend. Young children should not go on a food-restrictive diet, but you should start to encourage your son to eat food that is low in *Chemical Calories*. You should also start him on vitamin and mineral supplements specially formulated for children and essential fatty acids in the form of organic flax oil or fish oil that is free of pesticides and heavy metals. Shaklee's *Omega-3 Complex* is excellent for this purpose.

Children's vitamins often come in fun shapes or fruit flavors, but it can be much harder to get children to take flax or fish oil. If your child is not allergic to nuts, you can give him foods rich in essential fatty acids, such as walnuts or pumpkin seeds. Make sure your child also eats lots of soluble fiber from beans, oats, apples, or oranges, and gets more exercise. Together these steps should make a significant improvement in your child's weight problem.

Q. My teenage daughter has always struggled with her weight, but puberty is making the problem worse. Should she be starting on this program?

A. Puberty is a time when the body's hormones are going through a major upheaval. *Chemical Calories,* which have been linked with promoting early puberty in girls, can interfere with these hormones.[5] Although this book has been designed for adults, your daughter would definitely benefit from many of its principles. She should start by changing her diet to include food that is low in *Chemical Calories* and by taking vitamin and mineral, amino acid, and fatty acid supplements in doses suitable for her age.

This, with an increase in activity, should help her control her weight.

Weight problems can sometimes be exacerbated by puberty, as this life phase increases the need for certain nutrients to fuel adequate growth and sexual development.[6] Most of these nutrients, in particular vitamins A, D, B_6, and biotin, and zinc, calcium, magnesium, and essential fatty acids (particularly omega-3 fatty acids) are also used to power the *Slimming System*. As they are siphoned off to promote growth, few will be left for weight-control, and any shortage will exacerbate the weight gain as well as the other normal problems experienced during puberty, including acne and mood swings.

Q. I am an athlete, and though I don't want to lose weight, I do need to maximize my muscle strength. Could your program help me achieve this?

A. Absolutely. The program will increase the maximum extent to which your muscles will grow and improve your energy production. In other words, your muscle bulk will increase, along with your strength and endurance, which I imagine is just what you are looking for.

Q. I have just been through menopause and want to know if I can lose the excess weight I have gained.

A. Menopause causes a dramatic decline in natural estrogens and other slimming hormones in women, so after menopause the body is naturally "programmed" to gain a certain amount of weight. *Chemical Calories* accelerate and exacerbate these changes, contributing to "middle-age spread."[7] If you have never detoxed, the chances are that your buildup of *Chemical Calories* is quite substantial and that your *Slimming System* has been underperforming for some time. This program is for you and should help you lose the weight you have gained by providing your body with the essential nutrients you need in larger amounts at this time, namely, vitamins B, D, and E, calcium, zinc, magnesium, and omega-3 and omega-6 essential fatty acids. Another beneficial side effect is that your energy levels should greatly improve—which is always welcome!

Q. *My husband is very overweight, and our doctor has put him on a low-fat diet. We'd both like to follow your program, but most organic dairy foods seem to be full-fat. Is it more beneficial to buy organic products or low-fat products?*

A. Well, the best option is to try to find low-fat organic products. The next best would be to buy a low-fat product, as long as it is likely to be low in *Chemical Calories* (see Chapter 15).

Q. *I am getting alarmed at the size of my partner's pot belly, particularly since he has a family history of heart disease. Would he be able to lose his excess fat by going on this diet?*

A. From what you say, your partner would benefit enormously from this program. It will help shrink the fat deposits around his abdomen and potentially lower his risk of future heart disease on a number of different counts.

Q. *I'm confused by all the different labeling systems for meat and poultry. Some are free-range, some are organic, some non-GMO, and some are approved by animal welfare organizations. If I can't buy organic chicken, for example, will free-range chicken give me similar benefits?*

A. The short answer is no. Food can be labeled free-range if the animals have a certain amount of living space, but apart from that, their diets are similar to conventionally raised animals, and therefore they are exposed to the same chemicals. However, most organically raised chicken would pass as being free-range, due to generally higher standards for raising these animals.

Maximize Your Fitness:
How Exercise Revitalizes
Your *Slimming System*

I think, deep down, most of us already know that exercise has a whole host of health benefits. But to be more specific, exercise plays a major role in my program because it:

- Speeds up detoxification by mobilizing *Chemical Calories* from your fat. So exercise, in conjunction with the right supplement program, will speed up the rate at which you can detox.
- Increases your level of lean muscle tissue, so you will burn up more of your fat stores throughout the day.
- Boosts the levels of many of the most essential slimming hormones, including thyroid hormones, testosterone, and catecholamines.[1] This will increase your desire to exercise as well as improve the size, strength, and ability of your muscles to use up energy.

So it makes sense that if you are planning to start the diet, you will improve your figure much more quickly and effectively if you incorporate exercise as part of your program. There are many scientific reasons that this is in fact the case.

First, exercise, especially in short bouts, will lower your appetite, helping you stick to the diet.[2] Second, your mood will improve,[3] because exercise increases the levels of your natural mood-improving hormones. Third, exercise will greatly improve your figure, because it preserves and increases your lean muscle tissue.[4]

In addition, a certain degree of exercise will prevent the fall in metabolic rate that accompanies most food-restriction diets.[5] And, finally, an increased level of physical activity will also ensure that your skin remains firm and toned as you lose weight, so that not only will you look thinner, you also will look more fit and healthier.

Before plunging into exercise, however, you should check with your physician as to your activity level, especially if any of the following pertain to you: You have been physically inactive for six months or longer; you have a history of heart disease or high blood pressure; you have experienced dizziness, fainting, cold sweat, nausea, or uncomfortable pressure or chest pain; you have experienced chest pain radiating from chest to shoulders, neck, or arms; you have experienced shortness of breath; you have stomach or abdominal pain; you have difficulty breathing; you have experienced palpitations; you have asthma, emphysema, or lung disease; you have joint disease, such as arthritis, that might worsen with exercise; or you are an insulin-dependent diabetic.

A Regular Exercise Regime

Exercise can be broadly divided into two main categories: aerobic exercises, such as running or dancing, which improve your stamina and fitness rather than your muscle bulk, and resistance, or anaerobic, exercise, which is the kind used by bodybuilders to build muscle. Although both types of exercise are important, resistance exercise has the edge in enhancing your body shape and maintaining your muscle bulk when dieting.[6] Don't worry if you are not eager to go to a gym, as most forms of exercise are actually a mixture of aerobic and anaerobic activities.

To enhance your weight loss for the diet program, you will need to exercise for at least three thirty-minute sessions every week, to a level that will leave you out of breath or sweaty. Keep in mind that it is also important always to do that little bit extra every time you exercise, whatever you choose to do, so that you stimulate your muscles as well as the release of your slimming hormones.

There is really no preferred exercise; it could be weight training in the gym, swimming, or spring-cleaning the house. These will all help the *Slimming System,* so they are all equally acceptable. The trick is to find some kind of exercise that you really enjoy doing. Life is full of competing attractions, and you will only really stick to something that you enjoy. You should also try to vary your routine every few weeks to avoid getting bored. And it is important not to overdo things or use the gym equipment incorrectly, because that could lead to injury. If you attend a gym, always ask the instructors for advice on how to use the various machines and at what levels of difficulty you should use them.

Working Up to New Levels

To give you some ideas about the level of activity you need, I have divided a variety of activities into "light," "moderate," and "vigorous" categories. Ideally, you should be choosing moderate and vigorous activities for your thirty-minute sessions. However, if you have not previously been particularly active, you should start with light activities and work your way up as your fitness improves. One last thing: It is important to exercise for the full thirty minutes (or more) each time to get the maximum benefit from this program.

LIGHT ACTIVITIES

Table tennis, golf, social dancing and exercises (if not out of breath and sweaty), bowling, fishing, darts, pool, light gardening (weeding), or long walks at an average or slow pace.

MODERATE ACTIVITIES

Football, swimming, tennis, aerobics, cycling, table tennis, golf, social dancing and moderate exercises, heavy work activity (for example, mixing cement), heavy gardening (such as digging deep holes), heavy housework
(spring-cleaning), or long walks at a brisk pace.

VIGOROUS ACTIVITIES

Soccer, running (all forms), football, swimming, tennis, aerobics, rowing
vigorously, energetic social dancing, cycling, energetic exercising, hockey,
lacrosse, sawing wood, skiing energetically, skating energetically, some occupations that involve frequent climbing, lifting, or carrying heavy loads.

To help prevent injury, you should spend a few minutes warming up before you start your activity. After each session, you should make a note in
your diet diary of what type of activity you participated in, how you felt following each session, and how long you actually spent exercising.

If you ever work out in a gym, as I do, try to go on the running machine
when a good song comes on. This way, your mind is occupied listening to
the music or watching the video. Dancing is another excellent form of exercise and has the advantage of being a very social activity. And I always find
that time goes much faster if I work out to music.

Calories Burned per Fifteen Minutes of Activity	
ACTIVITY	CALORIES BURNED PER 15 MINUTES
Frisbee	53
Walking briskly (4 mph)	70
Bicycling (5.5 mph)	70

Golf	70
Dancing	80
Basketball, shooting baskets	80
Swimming	105
Hiking	105
Rowing	123
Jogging (9-minute mile)	193
Running (6-minute mile)	280

Top Tips for Detoxification

Exercise in itself is a wonderful way to detoxify, but there are a few extra things you can do to maximize the detox benefits from your sessions:

- Have a shower after a workout to wash off any toxic chemicals excreted onto your skin.
- Wipe away sweat during exercise to prevent reabsorption of toxins.
- Drink plenty of water before and after exercising to wash out lots of mobilized toxins.
- Take supplements to ensure that you soak up the *Chemical Calories* that you mobilize, and to minimize potential damage from free radicals.

At this point, you can see not only that exercise will enhance your *Slimming System* but also that keeping your *Slimming System* in shape will enhance your ability to exercise. So to make the most of the slimming benefits now available to you, all you need to do is get out of your chair and go for it!

Part Four

ACHIEVING A LIFESTYLE
THAT MINIMIZES
CHEMICAL CALORIES

18

Maintaining
the Slimmer New You

If you have been on the weight management program and have lost a significant amount of weight, then you have already accomplished a great deal. Congratulations! But no program would be complete without showing you how to maintain all the great progress you have made. The key to keeping that weight off is to continue to keep your body free of *Chemical Calories* by taking the essential supplements discussed in Chapter 15, maintaining a healthy diet, and continuing to engage in regular exercise.

Why You Need to Keep Taking Supplements

You might think that once you have achieved your ideal body weight, you won't need to keep taking supplements. You have to be philosophical here and accept that the whole world is so polluted that you cannot realistically prevent yourself from being exposed to *Chemical Calories*. By taking the supplements, you will be in a far better position to deal with the *Chemical Calories* that sneak past your defenses as well as the ones still lurking in your body. There is no way around it. Continuing to take the supplements will promote long-term health and well-being by protecting you against the development of chronic diseases and is vital in processing *Chemical Calories* and preventing those pounds from piling on again.

Increasing Food Intake to Maintain Weight Level

Unlike many weird and wonderful diets, the *Slimming System* program recommends the kinds of food that are the basis for your lifetime's eating habits after you come off the diet. But rather than stick to the quantities recommended in the weight loss diet, you can increase the total amount of food by approximately one-third.

Of course, people vary in size and shape, with some taller and more active men needing more food and some shorter and less active women needing less, but this plan provides an average level to aim for.

Eat Less Saturated Fat and Sugar

Some foods offer little or no benefit and just contain what are commonly described as "empty calories." This means that they add conventional calories but give the body or *Slimming System* few nutritional bonuses. In addition, the more of these foods you eat, the more slimming nutrients you will use up in processing them. So they are definitely not slimming friendly. Your goal should be to cut down on foods with high levels of saturated fat, sugary foods such as cakes, cookies, and candy, sauces laden with saturated fat, and fatty meats.

Change Your Eating Habits

Often, simple changes in your eating habits can make a very big difference in keeping your weight at its natural set point.

- Drink a glass of water a few minutes before a meal to take the edge off your hunger. And every day, drink at least eight eight-ounce glasses of filtered water.
- If hunger pangs strike, eat a piece of fruit or a pre-prepared raw vegetable.
- Eat slowly, giving your body sufficient time to register what you have just eaten.
- Listen to what your body needs, eat at the first signal of hunger, and stop when you are comfortable, not when you can't eat another bite.

If you follow this overall weight maintenance program, you are likely to find that your need for fatty or sweet foods will diminish naturally over time. This is because there will be fewer *Chemical Calories* to distort your appetite for fats and sugary carbohydrates. In addition, your *Slimming System* will have substantially repaired itself and will now be getting all the nutrients it needs to prevent the overwhelming need to eat certain foods, particularly fatty or sweet ones.

Keep Exercising!

Exercise is just as important in maintaining your new slimmer self as it is during the weight loss stage. It will help you keep unwanted pounds off, improve your sense of well-being, and reduce your overall risk of a host of weight-related diseases. And remember: People who keep exercising after they have lost weight are far more successful in keeping it off than people who fail to keep up their activity levels.

How to Avoid Relapses

After you have achieved your ideal weight, you should be very pleased with yourself, and why not? You'll look terrific and will have changed your life in an extremely positive way. At this point, you really do need to be careful. It's one thing to lose weight on a diet but quite another to keep weight off when you are not giving it your full attention.

As time goes on, you will need to stop and reconsider your situation. If you don't keep your exposure to *Chemical Calories* down and continue to take your supplements, your *Slimming System* will become damaged again, and you will start to put on weight again. The best thing to do in this case is to begin keeping a daily journal. It will help you to see if your food intake has risen too high and your intake of essential supplements has fallen too low. If you have regained more than just a couple of pounds, you could restart the Body Restoration Plan Diet. It may also be that you are still relatively contaminated with *Chemical Calories* and need to make further efforts to help your body get rid of them. So remember: All the information you need is in the earlier chapters.

Everything You Need for Success

You now have the information you need to eliminate *Chemical Calories* and the weight management and maintenance tools necessary to be successful in enhancing your health and happiness and in avoiding a substantial amount of future pain that would have been yours. Go for it. You deserve it!

19

Thirty Top Tips to Rid Your Life of *Chemical Calories*

To help you on your way to achieving the body of your dreams, here are thirty excellent ways to help rid your life of *Chemical Calories*. Every single one will help you detoxify and lose weight over the long term. And if you are just about to start the Body Restoration Plan Diet, they will help make your diet more effective.

The key is to do what you can when you can. While this might look like an awful lot of changes, the more you can cut out *Chemical Calories,* the slimmer you will eventually become. I've identified several products that can help you remove *Chemical Calories* from your environment. These products—like the dietary supplements I mentioned in Chapter 15—are distributed by Shaklee, and you can find out where to get them by visiting www.shaklee.com or by calling 1-800-742-5533.

None of these changes require you to give up any food; all they do is cut out the chemicals. This is, in effect, dieting without food restriction, which for many is a dream come true!

1. Reduce chemical contaminants in the air in your home and your office by using an air-cleaning system and by keeping your home well

ventilated. Remember that the air indoors tends to be far more polluted than it is outdoors (even in cities). Shaklee has an advanced
filterless air cleaner, *AirSource*® *3000*, which cleans 3,000 square
feet of air and reduces all three of the major forms of air pollution:
odors, microbes, and particulate matter.

2. Fill your rooms with plants that soak up airborne *Chemical Calories*.
   Spider plants are particularly useful—and can thrive without too
   much attention!

3. Wear disposable gloves and stand downwind of the vapors when re-
   fueling your car.

4. If you have highlights or other chemical treatments done at the
   beauty salon, take some extra vitamin C and E and a dose of soluble
   fiber supplements just before your visit. This will help protect your
   Slimming System from chemical damage, as sometimes a girl's got to
   do what a girl's got to do. Better still, see if they have a chemical-free
   alternative.

5. Always filter tap water before drinking it. Store filtered water in containers and keep them in a cool place, such as a refrigerator, to ensure purity and safety.

6. Install a household water filter to reduce the chemicals absorbed
   from bath or shower water.

7. When washing your hair, face, and body, use natural products with
   minimal chemicals, as they will be absorbed straight into your skin.
   Shaklee's *Enfuselle*® skin-care system includes gentle soap-free
   cleansers that gently remove dirt, makeup, and pollutants. Shaklee
   also has a remarkable patent-pending *ProSanté*™ system of hair-
   care products that removes pollutant buildup and protects your hair
   and scalp from environmental stresses.

8. Avoid skin-care products that are full of damaging chemicals. In addition to the cleansers, Shaklee's *Enfuselle* skin-care system includes products for individuals of all ages that have been designed
   to make the skin look and feel its youthful best. The cornerstone of
   the *Enfuselle* products is *Vital Repair+*®, a powerful antioxidant
   complex that breaks links in the chain of free-radical damage of the
   skin that is responsible for the loss of skin resiliency and firmness.

9. If you have clothes dry-cleaned, let them air outside or in a well-ventilated place for a day or two before putting them away in your closet.

10. Transform your bedroom into a *Chemical Calorie*–free oasis. Don't forget to keep your bedroom window slightly open at night if possible, but just to be on the safe side, make sure it has some sort of security lock.

11. Decorate your home with homegrown flowers rather than store-bought ones, which are likely to have been sprayed with pesticides.

12. If you have new appliances that have a strong odor, keep them in a well-ventilated room or outside (if appropriate) until the smell has mostly gone.

13. Don't heat foods, particularly fatty foods, in cling-film wraps.

14. If you do buy fatty foods (such as milk or cheese) in cling-film packaging, make sure you keep them at a low temperature in the fridge or freezer.

15. Try to avoid using those small portions of milk or cream in synthetic containers for your coffee or tea, particularly if they contain long-life products, since the longer the fatty fluids have been in contact with this flimsy synthetic material, the greater the potential contamination.

16. If you buy a new fridge, you can stop the synthetic chemical smell from being absorbed into your food by airing it outside with the door propped open until the smell subsides. Alternatively, if you have to use it immediately, you can make oil traps to soak up the odor as the material off-gasses. Fill a few small cups with any kind of vegetable oil, and leave them inside the fridge. Change the oil every few days until the smell disappears.

17. Take your supplements on a regular basis, as this is the key to long-term weight loss.

18. Never microwave or cook food in plastic containers, as higher temperatures enhance leaching of chemicals.

19. Don't drink boiling hot fluids from polystyrene cups. I know it can be tricky to keep to this one when at work or eating out, but it's worth asking if there is an alternative container. At work, you could

always bring in your own cup and supplies of organic coffee, tea bags, etc.

20. Be ruthless in throwing away all your unwanted polystyrene packaging or wrappings—this can be hard for natural hoarders, but do try!

21. When not in use, keep retained polystyrene boxes and packaging stored away in well-ventilated rooms.

22. Look for toys made from natural materials. They are safer for your child, and they will pollute the air inside the house less.

23. Use biodegradable and nontoxic cleaning products instead of chemicals to make your home sparkle. Shaklee, a pioneer in developing such products, offers a range of household products that contain no phosphates, no nitrates, and no corrosive chemicals, and that are designed to produce less packaging waste. Shaklee's *Basic-H®* is a biodegradable, highly effective all-purpose cleaner without caustic chemicals, odor, or toxic fumes that works fast to do hundreds of different jobs. When it's done, *Basic-H* degrades in the environment and breaks down into carbon dioxide and water to safely reenter the earth's ecosystem.

24. Make sure you rinse every trace of dishwashing liquid from your cutlery and dishes if you do use unnatural products. A better choice is to use environmentally friendly products such as Shaklee's *Satin Sheen®* dishwashing liquid and its phosphate-free *Basic-D®* automatic dishwashing concentrate.

25. Keep paints and solvents in a well-ventilated area as far away as possible from your living and sleeping space.

26. Safely dispose of all fly sprays, flea powders, and other synthetic pesticides. Try to find nontoxic alternatives—there are plenty out there. If you need a spray-on bug repellent, choose a natural remedy such as peppermint oil.

27. Go for the most environmentally friendly option when treating your home for bug infestations.

28. Try to avoid using synthetic-coated cooking utensils such as non-stick frying pans.

29. If you eat a meal that is high in *Chemical Calories*, take some soluble fiber as soon as possible, as this will greatly reduce the amount of *Chemical Calories* you will absorb from the meal. And if you plan

to eat out, why not just take the fiber in advance, as it will allow you to be more relaxed about what you eat.

30. If you spend a long time in the car, try to get an air filter, and keep a good distance away from the car in front of yours. This will allow the exhaust fumes to disperse before the air gets sucked into your car—as well as reduce your chances of an accident! Shaklee has developed a smaller *AirSource*® system that brings the technology and benefits of the *AirSource*® 3000 to your automobile.

20

Where Do We Go
from Here?

The conclusions from my own personal search for information about what makes us fatter, and what we can do about it, can be found in this book, which is the culmination of years of painstaking research. Personally, I have reaped a great deal of benefit from the research, since my weight now controls itself with little effort from me. In addition, my energy levels have shot up, and I am no longer plagued with coughs and colds. I hope that the same information about combating the fattening effects of toxic chemicals will now also revolutionize the lives of others.

I think by now you will have realized that my approach differs fundamentally from the old methods of dieting, which use simple food restriction alone. Dieting just by drastically cutting down what you eat is now in my belief virtually obsolete and could be downright dangerous in the twenty-first century. The evidence stacked up over the past fifty years shows this approach to be not only ineffective but also actually fattening over the long term, in addition to being a potentially significant cause of ill health.

For most of us, recognizing that we are contaminated with *Chemical Calories* will be the biggest step forward we can make. Once we accept this, it becomes much easier to understand why we gain weight and therefore why we need to protect ourselves against the re-release of chemicals as we lose weight.

The guidelines set out in these chapters describe a safe way in which we should now lose weight in our increasingly contaminated environment. For the first time ever, you have the power to control your own weight—by actively reversing the damage done by many years of chemical injury.

Blame Toxic Chemicals, Not Overweight People

What has motivated me all along this major journey of discovery has been a burning desire to help others control their weight. I know it sounds corny, but I get really upset when I see people suffer unnecessarily. That's probably what got me into medicine in the first place.

I don't for a single minute underestimate how much overweight people really can suffer. There's a powerful social stigma associated with being overweight, because it is widely assumed that it is the person's own fault. I hope the information I've gathered about toxic chemicals will help to get rid of that stigma.

In addition, there is a whole range of other disadvantages that come with being overweight, such as the relative lack of medical support. The medical establishment currently offers people relatively little active help and encouragement to solve their weight problems. I don't think this is malicious, though, but rather just a lack of understanding and minimal or no training in how to deal with the problem.

Happily, I have been able to move the finger of blame away from the individual and to point it at our increasing exposure to toxic chemicals. In the future, I hope that being overweight will be seen as a medical problem arising from a person's sensitivity to chemicals and specific nutritional deficiencies rather than as a condition that is the person's own fault. If I accomplish this, then all the hard work and effort I have put into researching and writing this book over the last few years will have been completely worthwhile.

The Headlines Once Again

Since my findings are so topical and groundbreaking, I expect them to trigger a much wider debate about chemicals and their many toxic effects. In my view, though, the more debate and research on this subject, the better. In order to bring things together, let's take a final look at the key issues raised throughout the book:

• The current fat epidemic is being caused to a large degree by the presence of toxic chemicals. Why? Because these toxic chemicals interfere with and damage the body's *Slimming System,* which humans have developed over millions of years in order to control their body weight. Damage to this system can result in an increased appetite, slower metabolism, reduced ability to burn off fat stores, and a reduced ability to exercise, all of which can actively promote weight gain.

• The way to lose weight permanently is by restoring and rejuvenating your *Slimming System.* You already have a highly developed system in place that is designed to promote weight loss. If you give your *Slimming System* what it needs to work properly and protect it from further damage, your body will become able to shift excess weight and keep it off by regulating your appetite, metabolism, and level of activity accordingly.

• What are *Chemical Calories,* and why are they so important? I have created a new unit known as a *Chemical Calorie* in order to estimate the fattening ability of all the different toxic chemicals we are now surrounded by. They are important because, by knowing which foods and nonfood products are low in *Chemical Calories,* we can be more selective in targeting the removal of those products that chemically appear to be the most fattening.

• A diet of processed foods has increased the severity of the fat epidemic. Processed foods tend to lack many of the vitamins, minerals, and crucial fats that are essential in powering the *Slimming System* and in ridding our bodies of toxic chemicals. So a diet of highly processed foods will result in higher body levels of *Chemical Calories* and therefore excess fat.

• The foods recommended on my program are *Slimming System*–friendly. In other words, they are high in slimming nutrients and low in

Chemical Calories. They make all the difference when it comes to keeping your *Slimming System* in excellent shape.

• Pesticides and other synthetic chemicals increase vitamin and mineral deficiencies. The presence of *Chemical Calories* in every aspect of our lives has permanently increased our body's need for certain nutrients. As a result, however good we may consider our diet to be, we all need to take nutritional supplements to ensure that our *Slimming System* is in full working order.

• Traditional dieting methods can make us fatter and damage our health. The way we need to diet has been permanently changed by the presence of toxic chemicals. Simple food restriction, with no consideration for the presence of *Chemical Calories,* releases high levels of toxins into the bloodstream from the body's fat stores. The resulting damage to the *Slimming System* and the rest of the body reduces our ability to lose weight and greatly increases our chance of developing a serious illness.

• However, given the right conditions, food-restriction dieting can be a great way to mobilize and rid our bodies of even the most persistent and hard-to-shift *Chemical Calories* with which we are now plagued.

• To maximize our ability to lose weight, we need to cut down our total exposure to *Chemical Calories*. Eating organic foods or foods low in *Chemical Calories,* in combination with lowering our exposure to *Chemical Calories* in our own environment, will significantly reduce the harm done to our *Slimming System*. As a result, our natural ability to burn up excess fat stores will be enhanced as our body's load of *Chemical Calories* is reduced.

• Your body's store of *Chemical Calories* must be safely removed to achieve maximum weight loss. The only effective way to remove many of the most highly fattening and persistent toxins is by consuming substances that bind to the chemicals, such as soluble fiber. These binding substances should be taken along with adequate nutrient supplementation, in order to enhance the body's natural detoxification system and protect the *Slimming System* from damage. Together, this will result in the safe removal of your lifetime's buildup of *Chemical Calories,* while minimizing any damage as a result of toxin mobilization.

• By optimizing your *Slimming System*, you will be enhancing the quality of your life. When you enhance your *Slimming System*, you will not just reduce your body fat; you also will effectively be reprogramming your body shape (by reducing the amount of fat and increasing the proportion of lean muscle), improving your health, and greatly enhancing your physical performance. In other words, by preventing the damage from toxic chemicals, you will be allowing your body to achieve its full potential.

The Effort Brings Rich Rewards

As we all know from experience, in order to achieve anything worthwhile in life, you have to make an effort. The same is true here. In order to gain these benefits, you will have to accept that you must make certain changes in how you shop for food, how you eat, and how you live. In addition, you will need to take quite a few supplements.

I admit this can't all be done overnight; it will take some time to implement all the necessary changes. For instance, depending on where you live, it might be either very easy or quite difficult to find organic produce or to get used to shopping with the benefit of the new *Chemical Calorie* charts. But as demand rises, these less polluted products will become more widely available, making it easier to keep your exposure to *Chemical Calories* as low as you can reasonably manage.

The beauty of this program is that you can actually lose weight by simple lifestyle changes that don't require any form of food deprivation at all. For example, just by filtering your household water or by using natural household cleaners, you can still lose weight. That realization is a true breakthrough.

And the more you achieve, the more you will find that your efforts are having a significant effect on your weight. This continual positive reinforcement will provide you with the encouragement you need to continue making lifestyle changes. I have seen the greatest skeptics totally converted into the most enthusiastic followers of this program because of the amazing results they have experienced.

One such skeptic, Jonathan Gold, began making various comments to his wife, Fiona, just after she went on the program. When she started to cut down on certain foods that are potentially high in *Chemical Calories,* such as salmon, he mentioned to her the changes he had noticed in her shopping habits. Salmon was one of his favorite foods, and he didn't look forward to cutting it out of his diet. After complaining bitterly about how he would never stop eating salmon and telling her how stupid she was to be following these "cranky" ideas, to prove his point he went out and bought a large quantity of it and proceeded to wolf it down during the Christmas and New Year holidays.

By chance, just as he finished the last mouthful, he found himself listening to a news item about how extremely polluted with highly toxic chemicals that have been strongly linked to cancer our salmon now is. She said that after a couple of days of similar stories in the press, he turned positively green and began to take a bit more interest in what my program was actually all about.

Not long after that, he started following the program himself. And although he never actively cut down the amount of food he consumed, after just a couple of months of cutting out *Chemical Calories* and taking the supplements, he discovered to his great delight that he had lost ten pounds totally effortlessly! His old suits began to fit again, and more and more people started commenting on his sleeker and healthier form. And to top it all, the severe symptoms of hay fever that had bothered him greatly for his entire adult life virtually disappeared.

Well, now he is totally over the moon with his new self and is a total convert to my program. And to his wife's constant amusement—given his initially strong negative attitude, owing to his lack of information—he now takes the lead in ensuring that the food he eats and the environment that surrounds him are kept as free of *Chemical Calories* as possible. This shows that there is nothing quite like experiencing these great benefits firsthand to provide a powerfully motivating force!

I feel extremely privileged to be able to present you with the means to achieve something that other weight loss programs have failed to achieve—permanent weight loss. I know from personal experience how much it has helped me, and I hope it will help you too. So with all my heart, I wish you good health and a very long and happy life.

Appendix A:
Common Toxic Chemicals

We are exposed to vast numbers of chemicals containing high levels of *Chemical Calories* in a huge number of everyday products. Although it would be impractical to go through all of them individually, I have selected some of the most common chemicals, just to highlight some of the places in which they can now be found in our food and environment.

The more you appreciate how widely these chemicals are used, and their individual longevity, the more clearly you will understand why we are now so contaminated with them.

ORGANOCHLORINES (AND OTHER ORGANOHALIDES)

What are they? Synthetically manufactured chemicals.
Examples: Organochlorine pesticides such as DDT, chlordecone, aldrin, dieldrin, endrin, toxaphene, heptachlor, lindane and its isomers, HCB (hexachlorobenzene); organochlorine pollutants such as dioxin, PCBs (polychlorinated biphenyls); organobromine fire retardants such as PBBs

(polybrominated biphenyls—used mainly in the United States) and PBDEs (polybrominated diphenyl ethers—used mainly in northern Europe).

Background information: Most developed countries have banned many types of organochlorine pesticides now, but owing to their previous extensive use and their long-lasting effects, their production is thought to have resulted in the permanent pollution of the entire planet. Moreover, these pesticides continue to be produced and used in developing countries, largely because of their relatively low cost, even though many of their dangers are well known. As contaminants, they accumulate up the food chain, and because of their high fat solubility and stability, they tend to concentrate in fatty tissues.

Compounds very similar to the organochlorine industrial chemicals (PCBs) and pesticides (DDT) are used as fire retardants. These substances, known as PBDEs and PBBs, are used extensively in developed and developing countries alike. These are also stable fat-loving chemicals that accumulate in fatty tissues and are nearly as toxic as their organochlorine counterparts.

Intended uses: General pesticides, common herbicides, insecticides, and fungicides; wood preservatives and treatment for termite protection; antimalaria spray; electrical conductors, fire retardants; paints and dyes, medicines.

Where they are found: As deliberately applied pesticide residues in food; as environmental contaminants in carnivorous fish, fatty meats, dairy products, human tissue, soil, water, and air adjacent to pollution sources; as contaminants in combusted leaded petrol; as contaminants in pesticides; as fire retardants on fabrics, clothes, curtains, furniture coverings, and wood; in electrical sealants, small capacitors, old refrigeration units, starter motors for fluorescent light switches; in carpets, carbonless duplicating paper, surface coatings, inks, and adhesives; in medicines such as nit shampoo and treatments for head and crab lice.

Estimated fattening ability: Extremely powerful, due to their extreme stability, our inability to expel them, and their widespread toxicity to the body's natural *Slimming System.*

ORGANOPHOSPHATES

What are they? Synthetically manufactured chemicals.

Examples: Organophosphate insecticides.

Background information: Organophosphates were originally created in 1845. Later, they were developed as a nerve gas and used in the Second World War. Since then, they have been used very extensively in many different areas of manufacturing, food production, and even medicine. They are now some of the most common pesticides detected on our foods.

Intended uses: Nerve gas in human warfare; pesticides for crops; sheep dips, cattle treatments, flea treatments for pets; wood infestation treatments; animal growth promoters; medicines, particularly treatments for lice, crabs, and nits; widespread industrial uses such as petrol additives, stabilizers in lubricating and hydraulic oils, synthetic additives, rubber additives, and flame retardants.

Where they are found: As pesticide residues in food, particularly on soft fruit, vegetables, and grain products; as pesticides used in agriculture; in household and garden pesticides such as fly spray; in pet treatments; on treated wood; as medicines; in car oil, petrol fumes, and rubber.

Estimated fattening ability: Organophosphates were previously used as animal growth promoters. Although not as fat-soluble and persistent as the organochlorine pesticides, they have different toxicities. They appear to be particularly damaging to the ability to exercise.

CARBAMATES

What are they? Synthetically manufactured chemicals.

Examples: Carbamate insecticides, dithiocarbamate fungicides, ETU (ethylenetiourea).

Background information: Action thought to be similar to that of organophosphates, but generally considered to be less toxic. Some effects last for a shorter period than those of organophosphates, but other toxic actions can last for much longer periods and result in permanent damage.

Intended uses: In pesticides such as insecticide, herbicide, fungicide, and antimicrobials; in treatments to prevent potatoes from sprouting and to rid livestock and chickens of parasites; in flea treatments for pets; in forestry and wood infestation treatments; as animal growth promoters; in manufacturing synthetic rubber; in other synthetics; as metal chelating agents.

Where they are found: In a wide range of foods and drinks, including potatoes, soybeans, citrus fruits, peanuts, tomatoes, beer and wine; in cigarettes and cigars; in cotton; in household and garden pesticides, including pet treatments, fly sprays, and mothballs; in treated wood; in water as contaminants; in medicines (see below).

Estimated fattening ability: Very powerful. Carbamates have been used as growth promoters in battery farm situations because of their ability to slow down the overall metabolic rate. They are used in medicine for their antithyroid hormone actions.

HEAVY METALS

What are they? Naturally occurring toxic metals.

Examples: Cadmium, lead, mercury, methyl mercury, tributyl tin (TBSPT).

Background information: These toxic substances occur naturally. However, due to their extensive industrial use, we are now being exposed to them at levels many times higher than those usually found in nature.

Intended uses: Industrial uses include use in pesticide formulations, electroplating, nickel plating, soldering, alloys, photoelectric cells, and storage batteries. Released in mining practices. Household uses include plumbing, building materials, cable covering, and paints; also used in dentistry, as petrol additives, and in insecticides.

Where they are found: As contaminants in drinking water and in food grown near roadsides. Found as human contaminants and is effluent in heavily polluted areas; used in amalgam fillings, crystal glass, petrol, batteries, roofing.

Estimated fattening ability: Moderate but their tendency to accumulate in the body over a number of years makes them very important.

SOLVENTS

What are they? Synthetically manufactured chemicals.

Examples: Organic solvents (styrene and polystyrene), chlorinated solvents (trichloroethylene), industrial solvents.

Background information: These chemicals are very widely used in a whole range of products. Certain liquid solvents, such as styrene, can be converted into polystyrene.

Intended uses: Solvents are used extensively throughout industry to dissolve or dilute oils and fats; as a petrol additive; as a major component of packaging and household materials; as a major substance in the dry-cleaning industry; in manufacturing synthetic rubbers, latex, and resins.

Where they are found: As synthetic fragrances in toiletries, detergents, skin-care products, perfumes, and aftershaves; in synthetic rubbers; as a heat-seal coating on metal foils (on yogurt and cream containers, etc.); as polystyrene cups and plates or polystyrene packaging; as a solvent for paints, in turpentine substitute, in shoe creams, floor waxes, and dyes; in household pesticides and medicines; as an environmental contaminant found in water, in the urban atmosphere, and in wildlife; in foods packaged in polystyrene; as a human contaminant; in glass fiber, petrol vapor, and exhaust fumes.

Estimated fattening ability: Moderate but still significant because of their very extensive presence in the environment. In particular, they appear to damage our slimming hormones.

Appendix B:
Your Ideal Body Weight
and Body Mass Index (BMI)

Years ago, we routinely determined our ideal body weight by looking at insurance company weight tables. Those tables were a good beginning but not particularly accurate because the ranges on them were so broad. Nowadays, the World Health Organization and the U.S. National Institutes of Health recommend using the Body Mass Index (BMI) to determine our ideal weight range, whether we are overweight, and, if so, to what extent.

Calculating BMI may at first appear difficult, but it is very easy. You can do it in a few brief steps. Just fill in the blanks below by answering the questions. You'll need a handheld calculator or pen and paper to do a little addition, multiplication, and division.

CALCULATE YOUR BMI

Your weight in pounds now is _____.
Your height in feet and inches is _____.

- Step 1: Convert your weight to kilograms by dividing your weight in pounds by 2.2:
  Your weight _____ ÷ 2.2 = _____ kilograms

- Step 2: Now convert your height to total inches by multiplying your height in feet by 12 inches:
  Height in feet × 12 inches = _____ + any remaining inches _____ = _____ total inches height

- Step 3: Convert your height in inches to meters by dividing the result of Step 2 by 40:
  Total inches in height _____ ÷ 40 = _____ total meters height

- Step 4: Square the height in meters by multiplying it by itself. In other words, multiply the result of Step 3 by itself like this:
  Total meters in height _____ × total meters in height _____ = _____ meters

- Step 5: Divide the weight in kilograms by the height in meters squared (divide the result of Step 1 by the result of Step 4):
  _____ kilograms of weight ÷ _____ meters = _____ = **BMI**

BMI Zones

BMI of 25 or less	Normal healthy range
BMI of 26	Overweight and flirting with danger
BMI of 27 to 29	Dangerously overweight
BMI of 30 or greater	Obese

Glossary of Terms

Adrenaline (epinephrine)   Stimulates heart rate, respiration rate, and metabolism. One of the most important slimming hormones we possess. It plays an important role in burning up excess fat and carbohydrates. Unfortunately, toxic chemicals very easily damage it.

Amino acids   The basic building blocks from which proteins are made up.

Antioxidants   Substances that are able to effectively neutralize and soak up harmful free radicals. Examples include vitamin A and beta-carotene, vitamins C and E, zinc, selenium, co-enzyme Q_{10}, and the amino acid glutathione.

Bioaccumulation   A buildup of chemicals that the body is unable to remove and thus ends up being stored.

Body weight set point   The weight (different for each individual) that the body tries to maintain through feast and famine.

Calorie   The energy needed to raise the temperature of 1 gram of water 1°C.

Calorific value   The amount of energy that the body can extract from a food.

Carbamates A class of very widely used pesticides that are added to food to kill fungus. They are used on a vast scale in agriculture and are commonly used in veterinary practice, in medicine, and as wood preservers.

Centigrade Now usually defined as 4.1868 joules.

Chemical Calories A *Chemical Calorie* is a measure of how damaging a toxic chemical is to the body's natural *Slimming System*. Foods high in *Chemical Calories* will be more chemically "fattening" than those low in *Chemical Calories*.

Chemical Calories rating A score allocated to particular chemicals indicating how toxic and damaging they are to the *Slimming System*. In practical terms, the higher the score a chemical possesses, the more fattening it will be.

Coenzyme Q_{10} This is a semiessential nutrient that plays a central role in boosting our energy levels. Like vitamins and minerals, it can be taken as a supplement.

Detoxification The removal of toxic substances from the body by the body's waste-disposal systems.

Estrogens A group of female hormones (also found in low levels in men) that promote female physical characteristics. Their decrease in women after menopause reduces the effectiveness of the *Slimming System*.

Free radicals These are highly damaging particles that are produced in cells by normal energy creation or by the detoxification of certain toxins. They are harmful because they damage and age all the tissues in which they are created. Pesticides, smoking, exhaust fumes, pollution, infections, burnt foods, fried foods, and sunburn increase the number of free radicals produced.

Fungicide A chemical that destroys fungus.

Glutathione An amino acid that is essential in breaking down toxic chemicals.

Growth promoter A chemical or substance that encourages growth in animals.

Herbicide A chemical that is toxic to plants and is commonly used as a weed killer.

Hormones Natural substances that act as natural internal chemical messengers in our bodies. They are released from one part of our bodies (glands) and are then carried around in the bloodstream to a tissue or organ that they then stimulate.

Insecticide A substance used to kill insects.

Insulin A hormone, the main role of which is to control our blood sugar levels. It also has a role in controlling our fat metabolism.

Metabolic rate The rate at which heat and other energy is produced and released from our bodies as a result of all the individual chemical reactions taking place.

Metabolism All the chemical reactions that occur within a living organism in order to maintain life.

Mineral A naturally ocurring inorganic substance needed by the human body in small quantities for good health.

Norepinephrine One of the most important slimming hormones we possess: As well as its role in powerfully suppressing our appetite, it is also absolutely essential in burning up excess body fat. Unfortunately, it is also exquisitely vulnerable to chemical damage.

Nutrient A substance that provides nourishment essential for the maintenance of life and growth.

Organic The term *organic* has three popular definitions, which causes a lot of confusion. The first definition includes the following: "natural plants and animals," "made from natural substances," or "allowed to grow naturally." People even talk about companies having organic growth, meaning gradual growth resulting from the hiring of employees as the company gains more business, as opposed to sudden growth resulting from the takeover of another company.

    The term is also used to describe food that is legally certified as organic. Organic food is supposed to have few added manufactured pesticides, antibiotics, hormones, and other additives, that is, meat, eggs, vegetables, and fruit produced without the use of artificial synthetic chemicals. The confusion created by these two definitions allows manufacturers to say that shampoo or other cosmetics are made from organic ingredients when they actually contain plant extracts that have been grown in a conventional way.

    And in the chemistry world, *organic* simply refers to any chemical with carbon and hydrogen in it. The study of organic chemistry is the study of compounds that contain carbon and hydrogen. Most pesticides and synthetic chemicals contain carbon, as they are often synthesized from petroleum or oil. So strictly speaking they are organic compounds, but unlike the substances they are derived from, they do not exist in nature.

Organic chemicals Substances derived from living organisms containing carbon and hydrogen.

Organic foods Food and other products grown, stored, preserved, and transported with minimal use of chemicals, and which tend to be less chemically contaminated than food produced using conventional means.

Organobromides A number of artificial and toxic compounds, which include the PBB and PBDE fire retardants. They are particularly persistent, fat soluble, and toxic. These substances tend not to be found in nature. And since they possess such a difficult molecular shape (because of the bromine component), our bodies' waste-disposal systems can find it very difficult to get rid of them.

Organochlorines A number of organic chemicals that contain the element chlorine. These types of compounds do not occur naturally, and due to our inability to remove them from our bodies—and their ability to accumulate in fatty tissues—they tend to be extremely persistent in the body as well as toxic. This varied group includes chemicals known as DDT, PCBs, and lindane.

Organophosphates Synthetic organic compounds that contain phosphorus, and which include highly toxic pesticides and nerve gases.

PBBs (polybrominated biphenyls) and PBDEs (polybrominated diphenyl ethers) Organic compounds that contain the element known as bromine. These substances are not usually found in nature and include a number of highly stable compounds that are particularly heat resistant—qualities that have led to their common use as fire retardants. However, due to our relative inability to remove them from our bodies, our bodily levels of these chemicals tend to accumulate throughout our lives.

PCBs (polychlorinated biphenyls) Although the manufacture of these types of organochlorines is now banned in most developed countries, these very stable organochlorines are still found in our environment as they are extremely persistent. They are also extremely persistent in our bodies.

Pesticide A substance used for destroying insects or other organisms harmful to cultivated plants or to animals and humans.

Plasticizers Chemicals added to plastics (synthetic resins) to produce or promote flexibility and to reduce brittleness.

Pollutants Substances that pollute or contaminate the environment, especially harmful chemical or waste material discharged into the atmosphere and water, including gases, particulate matter, pesticides, radioactive isotopes, sewage, organic chemicals and phosphates, solid waste, and many others.

Slimming System A set of highly evolved body functions that work together to bring about weight loss.

Supplement A substance taken to remedy dietary deficiencies.

Sympathetic nervous system (SNS) A specialized part of the body's nervous system that plays a key role in controlling body weight.

Synthetic chemical A man-made substance made by chemical synthesis, especially to imitate a natural product. These synthetic chemicals or substances do not exist in nature.

Testosterone A hormone that controls the development of male sexual characteristics. It is also very vulnerable to chemical damage.

Thermogenesis The production of heat in an animal or human. Many chemicals are able to reduce the body's ability to convert body fat stores into heat energy, so their net effect is the lowering of the body's temperature.

Thyroid hormones A group of hormones that regulate growth and development by altering the body's metabolic rate.

Vitamin Any of a group of compounds that are essential for normal growth and nutrition and are required in small quantities in a person's diet, because they cannot be created by the body.

Xenobiotics Foreign or unnatural compounds or chemicals (i.e., those that do not exist in nature).

Xenoestrogen A synthetic or phyto (plant) chemical not naturally found in the body that mimics the actions of natural estrogens (female hormones).

"Yo-Yo" dieting (or weight cycling) This is when people lose weight on a diet, then regain it when they have stopped dieting. They may repeat this pattern many times.

Resources

SLIMMING SYSTEMS LTD.

To help make it easier for people to follow the Body Restoration Plan Diet, Dr. Paula Baillie-Hamilton has founded the company Slimming Systems Ltd. Contact us at Slimming Systems Ltd. for the latest information on *Chemical Calories*, and please visit our website, www.slimmingsystems.com.

To find out more about Shaklee Corporation and its natural products, visit www.shaklee.com or call 1-800-742-5533.

Notes

INTRODUCTION: MAKING THE DISCOVERY

1. G. Gardner and B. Halweil, "Overfed and underfed: The global epidemic of malnutrition," *World Watch Paper* (2000)150: 7–11.

CHAPTER 1: THE FAT EPIDEMIC

1. G. Critser, "Let them eat fat: The heavy truths about American obesity," *Harpers, USA* April 2000.
2. Ibid.
3. Ibid.
4. M. S. Tremblay et al., "Secular trends in the body mass index of Canadian children," *Canadian Medical Association Journal* (2000), 163(11): 1429–33.
5. R. J. Kuczmarski et al., "Increasing prevalence of overweight among US adults," *Journal of the American Medical Association* (1994), 272(3): 205–11.
6. D. Collcutt and C. Evans, "Yes girls, it's true. You really are bigger these days," *Daily Mail,* London, 2 February 2000.
7. B. Marsh, "A two-inch pinch as men lose war of the waistline," *Daily Mail,* London, 15 June 2000.

8. A. G. Dulloo, "Regulation of body composition during weight recovery and thermogenesis," *Clinical Nutrition* (1997), 16(1): 25–35.

9. Ibid.

10. G. A. Colditz, "Economic costs of obesity," *American Journal of Clinical Nutrition* (1992) 55: 503s–7s.

11. L. Lissner et al., "Body weight variability in men: Metabolic rate, health and longevity," *International Journal of Obesity* (1990), 14(4): 373–83.

12. J. Baxter, "Obesity surgery—another unmet need," *British Medical Journal* (2000), 321(2): 523.

13. K. M. Flegal, "Overweight and obesity in the United States: prevalence and trends, 1960–1994," *International Journal of Obesity and Related Metabolic Disorders* (1998), 22(1): 39–47.

14. C. A. Dell et al., "Lipid and fatty acid profiles in rats consuming different high-fat ketogenic diets," *Lipids* (2001), 36(4): 373–8.

15. H. Tarnower and S. S. Baker, *The Complete Scarsdale Medical Diet* (London: Bantam Books, 1993).

16. B. Sears and B. Lawren, *Enter the Zone: A Dietary Road Map* (New York: Regan Books, 1995).

17. R. Atkins, *Dr. Atkins' New Diet Revolution* (New York: Avon Books, 1999).

18. R. B. Harris, "Role of set-point theory in regulation of body weight," *FASEB Journal* (1990), 415: 3310–18.

19. E. Alleva et al., "Statement from the work session on environmental endocrine-disrupting chemicals: neural, endocrine and behavioural effects," *Toxicology and Industrial Health* (1998), 14(1–2): 1–7.

20. U.S. Tariff Commission, "Synthetic Organic Chemicals," U.S. Government Printing Office, Washington, D.C., 1918–94.

CHAPTER 2: THE SYNTHETIC REVOLUTION

1. T. Colborn et al., "Environmental neurotoxic effects: the search for new protocols in functional teratology," *Toxicology and Industrial Health* (1998), 14(1/2): 9–23.

2. B. Holdsworth et al., *New Civil Engineer Supplement,* 25 September 2000.

3. D. V. Bailey, "Vyvyan Howard in bullet points," *Living Earth* (2001), 211(July–Sept.).

4. S. D. Stellman et al., "Relative abundance of organochlorine pesticides and polychlorinated biphenyls in adipose tissue and serum of women in Long Island, New York," *Cancer Epidemiology, Biomarkers & Prevention* (1998), 7: 489–96.

5. Center for Food Safety and Applied Nutrition, Office of Plant and Dairy Foods and Beverages, *Total Diet Study* (Rockville, MD: U.S. Food and Drug Administration, 2002), Market Basket 99-1.

6. P. Beaumont, "The chronic effects of pesticides," in *Pesticides, Policies and People: A Guide to the Issues* (London: Pesticides Trust, 1993), 83–92.

7. A. L. Rodrigues et al., "Effect of perinatal lead exposure on rat behaviour in open-field and two-way avoidance tasks," *Pharmacology and Toxicology* (1996), 79(3): 50–56.

8. U.S. Tariff Commission, "Synthetic Organic Chemicals."

9. S. Steingraber, *Living Downstream* (London: Virago Press, 1998): pp. 90–93.

10. Ibid.

11. J. A. Thomas and H. D. Colby (eds.), *Endocrine Toxicology* (Washington, D.C.: Taylor & Francis, 1996), p. 190.

12. L. E. Sever et al., "Reproductive and developmental effects of occupational pesticide exposure: the epidemiologic evidence," *Occupational Medicine* (1997), 12(2): 305–25.

13. K. Rozman et al., "Histopathology of interscapular brown adipose tissue, thyroid, and pancreas in 2,3,7,8-tetrachlorodibenzo-p-dioxin," *Toxicology and Applied Pharmacology* (1986), 82(3): 551–9.

14. J. R. Brown, "The effect of environmental and dietary stress on the concentration of 1,1-bis(4-chlorophenyl)-2,2,2,-trichloroethane," *Toxicology and Applied Pharmacology* (1970), 17: 504–10.

15. D. W. Nebert, "Human genetic variation in the enzymes of detoxification," in W. B. Jakoby, *Enzymatic Basis of Detoxification*, 1st ed. (Orlando: Academic Press, 1980), p. 32.

16. O. A. Iakovleva et al., "[Vitamin A and E allowance of the body in xenobiotic exposure]," *Voprosy Pitaniia* (1987), 3: 27–29.

17. R. W. Chadwick et al., "Effects of age and obesity on the metabolism of lindane by black a/a, yellow Avy/a, and pseudoagouti Avy/a phenotypes of (ys xvy) F1 hybrid mice," *Journal of Toxicology and Environmental Health* (1985), 16: 771–96.

18. C. Denzlinger et al., "Modulation of the endogenous leukotriene production by fish oil and vitamin E," *Journal of Lipid Mediators and Cell Signalling* (1995), 11(2): 119–32.

19. Center for Food Safety and Applied Nutrition, Office of Plant and Dairy Foods and Beverages, *Total Diet Study* (Rockville, MD: U.S. Food and Drug Administration, 2002), Market Basket 99-1.

20. Ibid.

CHAPTER 3: CHEMICALS THAT MAKE YOU FAT

1. J. Turner, "The welfare of broiler chickens—an analysis of the European Scientific Committee report of March 2000," Compassion in World Farming Trust, 2000.

2. J. F. Hancock, "Effects of estrogens and androgens on animal growth," in A. M. Pearson (ed.), *Growth Regulation in Farm Animals* (London: Elsevier Applied Science, 1991), p. 267.

3. T. Baptista et al., "Mechanism of the neuroleptic-induced obesity in female rats," *Progress in Neuro-Psychopharmacology and Biological Psychiatry* (1998), 22: 187–98.

4. J. Gawecki et al., "The effect of poisoning with dithane M-45 on oxygen uptake and energy balance in adult rats," *Acta Physiologica Polonica* (1976), 27(2): 169–74.

5. M. L. Trankina et al., "Effects of in vitro Ronnel on metabolic activity in subcutaneous adipose tissue and skeletal muscle from steers," *Journal of Animal Science* (1985), 60(3): 652–8.

6. U.S. Tariff Commission, "Synthetic Organic Chemicals"; K. M. Flegal, "Overweight and obesity in the United States."

7. K. M. Flegal, "Overweight and obesity in the United States: prevalence and trends, 1960–1994."

8. S. D. Stellman et al., "Adipose and serum levels of organochlorinated pesticides and PCB residues in Long Island women: Association with age and body mass," *American Journal of Epidemiology* (1997), SER Abstract S21, p. 81.

9. J. Ashby et al., "Lack of effects for low dose levels of bisphenol A and diethylstilbestrol on the prostate gland of CFI mice exposed in utero," *Regulatory Toxicology and Pharmacology* (1999), 30(2, pt. 1): 156–66.

10. B. D. Hardin et al., "Evaluation of 60 chemicals in a preliminary developmental toxicity test," *Carcinogens, Mutagens and Teratogens* (1987), 7: 29–48.

11. D. R. Clark, "Bats and environmental contaminants: A review," U.S. Department of the Interior: Fish and Wildlife Service, Special Scientific Report, Washington, D.C., *Wildlife* No. 235 (1981): 1–29.

12. K. Takahama et al., "Toxicological studies on organochlorine pesticides: 1. Effect of long term administration of organochlorine pesticides on rabbit weight and organ weight," *Nippon Hoigaku Zasshi* (1972), 26(1): 5–10.

13. J. C. Lamb et al., "Reproductive effects of four phthalic acid esters in the mouse," *Toxicology and Applied Pharmacology* (1987), 88(2): 255–69.

14. Ashby et al., "Lack of effects for low dose levels of bisphenol A and diethylstilbestrol."

15. Trankina et al., "Effects of in vitro Ronnel."

16. J. E. Morley, "Anorexia in older persons," *Epidemiology* (1996), 8(2): 134–55.

17. P. B. Kaplowitz and S. Jennings, "Enhancement of linear growth and weight gain by cyproheptadine in children with hypopituitarism receiving growth hormone therapy," *Journal of Pediatrics* (1987), 110(1): 140–43.

18. M. T. Antonio et al., "Neurochemical changes in newborn rat's brain after gestational cadmium and lead exposure," *Toxicology Letters* (1999), 104(1–2): 1–9.

19. E. A. Field et al., "Developmental toxicology evaluation of diethyl and dimethyl phthalate in rats," *Teratology* (1993), 48(1): 33–44.

20. B. N. Gupta et al., "Effects of a polybrominated biphenyl mixture in the rat and mouse: I. Six-month exposure," *Toxicology and Applied Pharmacology* (1983), 68(1): 1–18.

21. Trankina et al., "Effects of in vitro Ronnel."

22. J. L. De Bleecker et al., "Neurological aspects of organophosphate poisoning," *Clinical Neurology and Neurosurgery* (1992), 94: 93–103.

23. S. F. Ali et al., "Effect of an organophosphate (Dichlorvos) on open field behaviour and locomotor activity: correlation with regional brain monoamine levels," *Psychopharmacology* (1980), 68(1): 37–42.

24. J. T. Yen et al., "Effect of carbadox on growth, fasting metabolism, thyroid function and gastrointestinal tract in young pigs," *American Institute of Nutrition* (1984), 115: 970–79.

25. T. Tanaka, "Reproductive and neurobehavioural effects of chlorpropham administered to mice in the diet," *Toxicology and Industrial Health* (1997), 13(6): 715–26.

26. A. Heeremans et al., "Elimination profile of methylthiouracil in cows after oral administration," *Analyst* (1998), 123: 2625–8.

27. A. L. Sawaya and P. G. Lunn, "Lowering of plasma triiodothyronine level and sympathetic activity does not alter hypoalbuminaemiain rats fed a low protein diet," *British Journal of Nutrition* (1998), 79(5): 455–62.

28. K. J. Van den Berg et al., "Interactions of halogenated industrial chemicals with transthyretin and effects of thyroid hormone levels in vivo," *Archives of Toxicology* (1991), 65: 15–19.

29. A. Vigano et al., "Anorexia and cachexia in advanced cancer patients," *Cancer Surveys* (1994), 21: 99–115.

30. M. C. Nesheim, "Some observations on the effectiveness of anabolic agents in increasing the growth rate of poultry," *Environmental Quality and Safety. Supplement* (1976), 5: 110–14.

31. J. S. Cranmer and D. L. Avery, "Postnatal endocrine dysfunction resulting from prenatal exposure to carbofuran, diazinon or chlordane," *Journal of Environmental Pathology and Toxicology* (1978), 2: 375–67.

32. J. F. Hancock, "Effects of estrogens and androgens on animal growth," p. 271.

33. V. W. Hays, "Effect of antibiotics," in Pearson (ed.), *Growth Regulation in Farm Animals,* pp. 299–320.

34. Ibid.

35. Vigano et al., "Anorexia and cachexia."

36. S. H. Kennedy and D. S. Goldbloom, "Current perspectives on drug therapies for anorexia nervosa and bulimia nervosa," *Practical Therapeutics* (1991), 41(3): 367–77.

37. Ibid.

38. Morley, "Anorexia in older persons."

39. E. M. Walker, Jr. et al., "Prevention of cisplatin-induced toxicology by selected dithiocarbamates," *Annals of Clinical and Laboratory Science* (1994), 24(2): 121–33.

40. E. Van Ganse et al., "Effects of antihistamines in adult asthma: a meta-analysis of clinical trials," *European Respiratory Journal* (1997), 10(10): 2216–24.

41. Bailey, "Vyvyan Howard in bullet points."

42. Alleva et al., "Statement from the work session on environmental endocrine-disrupting chemicals."

43. Nebert, *Human Genetic Variation,* p. 32.

44. W. B. Deichmann et al., "Effects of starvation in rats with elevated DDT and dieldrin tissue levels," *Internationales Archiv für Arbeitsmedizin* (1972), 29: 233–52.

45. R. W. Chadwick et al., "Possible antiestrogenic activity of lindane in female rats," *Journal of Biochemical Toxicology* (1988), 3: 147–58.

46. Center for Food Safety and Applied Nutrition, Office of Plant and Dairy Foods and Beverages, *Total Diet Study* (Rockville, MD: U.S. Food and Drug Administration, 2002), Market Basket 99-1.

47. Ibid.

48. D. C. Villeneuve et al., "Effect of food deprivation on low level hexachlorobenzene exposure in rats," *Science of the Total Environment* (1977), 8(2): 179–86.

49. Stellman et al., "Adipose and serum levels."

50. M. E. Hovinga, et al., "Environmental exposure and lifestyle predictors of lead, cadmium, PCB, and DDT levels in Great Lakes fish eaters," *Archives of Environmental Health* (1993), 48: 98–104.

51. I. Tsuritani et al., "Polymorphism in ALDH2–genotype in Japanese men and the alcohol–blood pressure relationship," *American Journal of Hypertension* (1995), 8(11): 1053–9.

52. Chadwick et al., "Effects of age and obesity."

53. M. E. Hovinga, et al., "Environmental exposure and lifestyle predictors."

54. F. P. Guengerich, "Influence of nutrients and other dietary materials on cytochrome P-450 enzymes," *American Journal of Clinical Nutrition* (1995), 61(3): 651s–658s.

55. J. M. Schildkraut et al., "Environmental Contaminants and body fat distribution," *Cancer Epidemiology, Biomarkers & Prevention* (1999), 8: 179–83.

56. Schildkraut et al., "Environmental contaminants."

CHAPTER 4: YOUR NATURAL *SLIMMING SYSTEM*

1. Harris, "Role of set-point theory."

2. C. Michel and M. Cabanac, "Effects of dexamethasone on the body weight set point of rats," *Physiology and Behavior* (1999), 68(1–2): 145–50.

3. R. E. Keesey and M. D. Hirvonen, "Body weight set-points: determination and adjustment," *Journal of Nutrition* (1997), 127(9): 1875s–1883s.

4. M. E. Hadley, *Endocrinology,* 3rd ed. (Englewood, NJ: Prentice-Hall International [Publishers], 1992), pp. 19–21.

5. Ibid., pp. 362–90.

6. K. D. Brownell and C. G. Fairburn (eds.), *Eating Disorders and Obesity: A Comprehensive Handbook* (New York: Guilford Press, 1995), pp. 3–7.

7. J. Clarke, *Body Foods for Life* (London: Weidenfeld & Nicolson, 1998), p. 200.

8. Harris, "Role of set-point theory."

9. P. Bjorntorp, "Endocrine abnormalities of obesity," *Metabolism* (1995), 44 [9 (suppl. 3)]: 21–23.

10. P. T. Williams, "Weight set-point theory predicts HDL-cholesterol levels in previously obese long-distance runners," *International Journal of Obesity* (1990), 14(5): 421–7.

11. Y. Hu et al., "Comparisons of serum testosterone and corticosterone between exercise training during normoxia and hypobaric hypoxia in rats," *European Journal of Applied Physiology* (1998), 78: 417–21.

12. S. V. Roberts et al., "Energy expenditure and intake in infants born to lean and overweight mothers," *New England Journal of Medicine* (1988), 318: 461.

13. T. Archer and A. Fredriksson, "Functional changes implicating dopaminergic systems following perinatal treatments," *Developmental Pharmacology and Therapeutics* (1992), 18(3–4): 201–2.

14. J. A. Levine et al., "Role of non-exercise activity thermogenesis in resistance to fat gain in humans," *Science* (1999), 283 (5399): 212–14.

15. D. S. Miller and P. Mumford, "Obesity: physical activity and nutrition," *Proceedings of the Nutritional Society* (1966), 25(2): 100–107.

16. R. Scott Van Zant, "Influence of diet and exercise on energy expenditure—a review," *International Journal of Sport Nutrition* (1992), 2: 1–19.

17. C. Bouchard et al., "Genetic effect in resting and exercise metabolic rates," *Metabolism* (1989), 38: 364.

18. L. Landsberg et al., "Sympathoadrenal system and regulation of thermogenesis," *American Journal of Physiology* (1984), 247(2, pt. 1): E181–9.

19. G. R. Goldberg et al., "Longitudinal assessment of the components of energy balance in well-nourished lactating women," *American Journal of Clinical Nutrition* (1991), 54: 788–98.

20. A. G. Dulloo and D. S. Miller, "The effect of parasympathetic drugs on energy expenditure: Relevance to the autonomic hypothesis," *Canadian Journal of Physiology and Pharmacology* (1986), 64: 586–91.

21. R. T. Jung et al., "Reduced thermogenesis in obesity," *Nature* (1979), 279: 322–3.

22. B. Zahorska-Markiewicz, "Thermic effect of food and exercise in obesity," *European Journal of Applied Physiology* (1980), 44: 231–5.

23. Ali et al., "Effect of an organophosphate (Dichlorvos)."

24. A. Moor de Burgos et al., "Blood vitamin and lipid levels in overweight and obese women," *European Journal of Clinical Nutrition* (1992), 46: 803–8.

25. S. Klaus, "Functional differentiation of white and brown adiposities," *Bioessays* (1997), 19(3): 215–23.

26. Moor de Burgos et al., "Blood vitamin and lipid levels."

27. R. S. Strauss, "Comparison of serum concentrations of alpha-tocopherol and beta-carotene in a cross-sectional sample of obese and non-obese children (NHANES III). National Health and Nutrition Examination Survey," *Journal of Pediatrics* (1999), 134(2): 160–5.

28. G. J. Naylor et al., "A double blind placebo controlled trial of ascorbic acid in obesity," *Nutrition and Health* (1985), 4(1): 25–28.

29. Gardner and Halweil, "Overfed and underfed."

30. M. Ohrvall et al., "Lower tocopherol serum levels in subjects with abdominal adiposity," *Journal of Internal Medicine* (1993), 234(1): 53–60.

31. R. B. Singh et al., "Association of low plasma concentrations of antioxidant vitamins, magnesium and zinc with high body fat percent measured by bioelectrical impedance analysis in Indian men," *Magnesium Research* (1998), 11(1): 3–10.

CHAPTER 5: HOW CHEMICALS MAKE YOU FAT

1. H. D. Colby et al., "Toxicology of the adrenal cortex: Role of metabolic activation," in J. A. Thomas and H. D. Colby, eds., *Endocrine Toxicology*, 2nd ed. (Washington, D.C.: Taylor and Francis, 1997), pp. 81–131.

2. W. Rea, "Nervous system," in *Chemical Sensitivity*, vol. 3 (Boca Raton, FL: Lewis Publishers, 1995), pp. 1727–885.

3. M. B. Abou-Donia and D. M. Lapadula, "Mechanisms of organophosphorus ester-induced delayed neurotoxicity: Type I and type II," *Annual Review of Pharmacology and Toxicology* (1990), 30: 405–40.

4. N. C. Rawlings et al., "Effects of the pesticides carbofuran, chlorpyrifos, dimethoate, lindane, triallate, trifluralin, 2,4–D, and pentachlorophenol on the metabolic endocrine and reproductive endocrine system in ewes," *Journal of Toxicology and Environmental Health* (1998), 54(Part A): 21–36.

5. M. J. DeVito and L. S. Birnbaum, "Dioxins: Model chemicals for assessing receptor-mediated toxicity," *Toxicology* (1995) 102: 115–23; G. Cehovic et al., "Paraxon: Effects on rat brain cholinesterase and on growth hormone and prolactin of pituitary," *Science* (1972), 175: 1256–8.

6. J. A. Richardson et al., "Catecholamine metabolism in humans exposed to pesticides," *Environmental Research* (1975), 3(9 June): 290–94.

7. Colby et al., "Toxicology of the adrenal cortex."

8. J. R. Beach et al., "Abnormalities on neurological examination among sheep farmers exposed to organophosphorous pesticides," *Occupational and Environmental Medicine* (1996), 53: 520–25.

9. T. Namba et al., "Poisoning due to organophosphate insecticides," *American Journal of Medicine* (1971), 50: 475–92.

10. R. J. Zwiener and C. M. Ginsburg, "Organophosphate and carbamate poisoning in infants and children," *Pediatrics* (1988), 81(5), 683.

11. Iakovleva et al., "[Vitamin A and E allowance]."

12. E. J. Cheraskin, "Antioxidants in health and disease," *Journal of the Optometric Association* (1996), 67(1): 50–57.

13. P. Holford, "The myth of the well-balanced diet," in *The Optimum Nutrition Bible* (London: Piatkus, 1999), pp. 27–33.

14. Field et al., "Developmental toxicology evaluation."

15. Vigano et al., "Anorexia and cachexia."

16. R. Husain et al., "Differential responses of regional brain polyamines following in utero exposure to synthetic pyrethroid insecticides: a preliminary report," *Bulletin of Environmental Contamination and Toxicology* (1992), 49(3): 402–9.

17. Gawecki et al., "The effect of poisoning with dithane M-45."

18. K. N. Chetty et al., "Effect of cadmium on ATPase activities in rats fed on iron-deficient and sufficient diets," *Journal of Environmental Science and Health* (1980), 15(4): 379–93.

19. Cehovic et al., "Paraxon."

20. Guengerich, "Influence of nutrients."

21. W. B. Deichmann et al., "Dieldrin and DDT in the tissues of mice fed aldrin and DDT for seven generations," *Archives of Toxicology* (1975), 34(3): 173–82.

22. P. D. Hrdina et al., "Role of norepinephrine, 5–hydroxytryptamine and acetylcholine in the hypothermic and convulsive effects of alpha-chlordane in rats," *European Journal of Pharmacology* (1974), 26(2): 306–12.

23. Richardson et al., "Catecholamine metabolism."

24. W. Rea, "Nutritional status and pollutant overload," in *Chemical Sensitivity*, vol. 1 (Boca Raton, FL: Lewis Publishers, 1992), pp. 395–6.

25. Deichmann et al., "Dieldrin and DDT."

26. Nebert, *Human Genetic Variation*, p. 32.

27. Chadwick et al., "Effects of age and obesity."

28. Holford, "The myth of the well-balanced diet."

29. J. To-Figueras et al., "Mobilization of stored hexachlorobenzene and p,p-dichlorodiphenyldichloroethylene during partial starvation in rats," *Toxicology Letters* (1988), 42(1): 79–86.

30. S. N. Blair et al., "Body weight change, all-cause mortality, and cause-specific mortality in the multiple risk factor intervention trial," *Annals of Internal Medicine* (1993), 119[7 (part 2)]: 749–57.

CHAPTER 6: ALL ABOUT *CHEMICAL CALORIES*

1. Harris, "Role of set-point theory."

2. A. C. Casey et al., "Aroclor 1242 inhalation and ingestion by Sprague-Dawley rats," *Journal of Toxicology and Environmental Health* (1999), 56(5): 311–42.

3. Gupta et al., "Effects of a polybrominated biphenyl mixture in the rat and mouse."

4. Chetty et al., "Effect of cadmium on ATPase."

5. I. Chu et al., "Long-term toxicity of octachlorostyrene in the rat," *Fundamental and Applied Toxicology* (1986), 6(1): 69–77.

6. V. C. Moser et al., "A multidisciplinary approach to toxicological screening: III. Neurobehavioural toxicology," *Journal of Toxicology and Environmental Health* (1995) 45(2): 173–210.

7. Center for Food Safety and Applied Nutrition, Office of Plant and Dairy Foods and Beverages, *Total Diet Study* (Rockville, MD: U.S. Food and Drug Administration, 2002), Market Baskets 98-2, 98-3, 98-4, 99-1

CHAPTER 7: WHAT MAKES STRAWBERRIES MORE "FATTENING" THAN AVOCADOS?

1. Center for Food Safety and Applied Nutrition, Office of Plant and Dairy Foods and Beverages, *Total Diet Study* (Rockville, MD: U.S. Food and Drug Administration, 2002), Market Baskets 98-2, 98-3, 98-4, 99-1.

2. B. J. Liska and W. J. Stadelman, "Effects of processing on pesticides in foods," *Residue Reviews* (1969), 29: 61–72.

3. J. E. Bjerk and E. M. Brevik, "Organochlorine compounds in aquatic environments," *Archives of Environmental Contamination and Toxicology* (1980), 9(6): 743–50.

4. Trankina et al., "Effects of in vitro Ronnel."

5. P. M. Friar and S. L. Reynolds, "The effect of home processing on post-harvest fungicide residues in citrus fruit," *Food Additives and Contaminants* (1994), 11(1): 57–70.

CHAPTER 8: DON'T PANIC, GO ORGANIC

1. B. P. Baker et al., "Pesticide residues in conventional, integrated pest management (IPM) grown and organic foods: Insight from three US data sets," *Food Additives and Contaminants* (2002), 19(5): 427–46.

2. V. Worthington, "Effect of agricultural methods on nutritional quality: A comparison of organic with conventional crops," *Alternative Therapies* (1998), 4(1): 58–69.

3. S. S. Schiffman et al., "Environmental pollutants alter taste responses in the gerbil," *Pharmacology, Biochemistry and Behavior* (1994), 52(1): 189–94.

4. A. Mayer, "Historical changes in the mineral content of fruits and vegetables," *British Food Journal* (1997), 99(6): 207–11.

5. V. Worthington, "Nutritional quality of organic versus conventional fruits, vegetables, and grains," *Journal of Alternative and Complementary Medicine* (2001), 7(2), 161–73.

6. J. B. Pangborn and B. Smith, "Elemental content of some organic foods vs. commercial foods," presented at the 13th Annual International Symposium on Man and his Environment in Health and Disease, Dallas, TX, 1995.
7. Ibid.

CHAPTER 9: EATING FEWER *CHEMICAL CALORIES*

1. M. E. Zabik and R. Schemmel, "Influence of diet on hexachlorobenzene accumulation in Osborne Mendel rats," *Journal of Environmental Pathology and Toxicology* (1980), 4(5–6): 97–103.
2. H. J. Schattenberg, 3rd et al., "Effect of household preparation on levels of pesticide residues in produce," *Journal of AOAC International* (1996), 79(6): 1447–53.
3. Friar and Reynolds, "The effect of home processing."
4. J. C. Street, "Methods of removal of pesticide residues," *Canadian Medical Association Journal* (1969), 100: 154–60.
5. Ibid.
6. Liska and Stadelman, "Effects of processing."
7. Friar and Reynolds, "The effect of home processing."
8. D. D. Hemphill et al., "Effect of washing, trimming and cooking on levels of DDT and derivatives in green beans," *Journal of Agricultural and Food Chemistry* (1967), 15: 290.
9. Parents for Safe Food and Friends of the Earth, "Dangerous Agrochemicals in Supermarket Foods," Parents for Safe Food and Friends of the Earth press release, UK, 14 February 1990.
10. A. Schecter et al., "A comparison of dioxins, dibenzofurans and coplanar PCBs in uncooked and broiled ground beef, catfish, and bacon," *Chemosphere* (1998), 37(9–12): 1723–30.
11. M. D. Rose et al., "The effect of cooking on veterinary drug residues in food: Ivermectin," *Food Additives and Contaminants* (1998), 15(2): 157–61.

CHAPTER 10: PURE WATER, YOUR WEIGHT-LOSS FRIEND

1. L. McTaggart, "Assault on a generation," *What Your Doctor Doesn't Tell You* (2000), 11(6): 5.
2. J. M. Esch, "Hydrological Investigation, Nottawa Sepee Site, Village of Napoleon, Jackson County," Michigan Department of Natural Resources, 1995.
3. M. A. Medinsky et al., "Effects of a thirteen-week inhalation exposure to ethyl tertiary butyl ether on Fischer-344 rats and CD-1 mice," *Toxicological Science* (1999), 51(1): 108–18.

4. K. Cooke and M. H. Gould, "The health effects of aluminium—a review," *Journal of the Royal Society of Health* (1991), 111(5): 163–68.
5. W. Rea, "Avoidance-Water," in *Chemical Sensitivity*, vol. 4, (Boca Raton, FL: Lewis Publishers, 1996), pp. 2359–82.
6. A. L. Gittleman, "Water: The Chlorine Connection," *The Living Beauty Detox Program*, (San Francisco: HarperCollins, 2000).
7. S. Clark, "Water, the drink of life," *The Times 2 Alternative Health*, London, 21 March 2000.
8. S. Welle et al., "Increased plasma norepinephrine concentrations and metabolic rates following glucose ingestion in man," *Metabolism* (1980), 29(9): 806–9.

CHAPTER 11: *CHEMICAL CALORIES* LURK
ALL AROUND YOU

1. G. M. Currado and S. Harrad, "The significance of indoor air inhalation as a pathway of human exposure to PCBs," *Organohalogen Compounds* (1997), 33: 377–81.
2. R. P. Benedetti, "Understanding fire retardant and flame resistant materials," *Journal of the American College Health Association* (1979), 27(6): 311–41.
3. K. Nesaretnam et al., "3,4,3',4'-Tetrachlorobiphenyl acts as an estrogen in vitro and in vivo," *Molecular Endocrinology* (1996), 10: 912–36.
4. H. M. Haynes et al., "Case control study of canine malignant lymphoma: Positive association with dog owners use of 2,4–D," *Journal of the National Cancer Institute* (1991), 83: 1226–31.
5. M. Levy, "Dental Amalgam: toxicological evaluation and health risk assessment," *Journal of the Canadian Dental Association* (1995), 61(8): 667–8, 671–4.

CHAPTER 12: BEATING THE *CHEMICAL CALORIE*

1. P. Dingle et al., "Reducing formaldehyde exposure in office environments using plants," *Bulletin of Environmental Contamination and Toxicology* (2000), 64(2): 302–8.
2. A. Clarke et al., "Organic home," in *Living Organic: Easy steps to an organic family lifestyle* (London: Time-Life Books, 2001), p. 98.

279

CHAPTER 13: REPAIR AND REVITALIZE YOUR
NATURAL *SLIMMING SYSTEM*

1. C. S. Hun et al., "Increased uncoupling protein2 mRNA in white adipose tissue, and decrease in leptin, visceral fat, blood glucose, and cholesterol in KK-Ay mice fed with eicosapentaenoic and docosahexaenoic acids in addition to linolenic acid," *Biochemical and Biophysical Research Communications* (1999), 259(1): 85–90.

2. G. V. Skuladottir and M. Johannsson, "Inotropic response of rat heart papillary muscle to alpha 1– and beta-adrenoceptor stimulation in relation to dietary n-6 and n-3 polyunsaturated fatty acids (PUFA) and age," *Pharmacology and Toxicology* (1997), 80(2): 85–90.

3. T. Horie et al., "Docosahexaenoic acid exhibits a potent protection of small intestine from methotrexate-induced damage in mice," *Life Science* (1998), 62(15): 1333–8.

4. S. M. Watkins et al., "DHA reduces free radicals generation in the fetal rat brain," *Journal of Lipid Research* (1998), 39(8): 1583–8.

5. A. P. Simopoulous, "Omega-3 fatty acids in health and disease and in growth and development," *American Journal of Clinical Nutrition* (1991), 54(3): 438–63.

6. M. N. Jacobs, "Organochlorine residues in fish oil dietary supplements: Comparison with industrial grade oils," *Chemosphere* (1998), 37(9–12): 1709–21.

7. L. H. Garthoff et al., "Blood chemistry alterations in rats after single and multiple gavage administration of polychlorinated biphenyl," *Toxicology and Applied Pharmacology* (1981), 60(1): 33–44.

8. Ibid.

9. P. Pittet et al., "Thermic effect of glucose in obese subjects studied by direct and indirect calorimetry," *British Journal of Nutrition* (1976), 35: 281.

10. Ibid.

11. Zabik and Schemmel, "Influence of diet on hexachlorobenzene accumulation."

12. Guengerich, "Influence of nutrients."

13. W. Rea, "Nutritional status and pollutant overload," in *Chemical Sensitivity*, vol. 1 (Boca Raton, FL: Lewis Publishers, 1992): pp. 345–93.

14. Ibid.

15. G. Y. Nicolau, "Circadian rhythms of RNA, DNA and protein in the rat thyroid, adrenal and testis in chronic pesticide exposure: II. Effect of the herbicides, aminotriazole and alachlor," *Endocrinologie* (1983), 21(2): 105–12.

16. Rea, "Nutritional status and pollutant overload."

17. J. C. Street and R. W. Chadwick, "Ascorbic acid requirements and metabolism in relation to organochlorine pesticides," *Annals of the New York Academy of Sciences* (1975), 258(30 September): 132–43.

18. Rea, "Nutritional status and pollutant overload."

NOTES

CHAPTER 14: SHED YOUR BODY STORES
OF *CHEMICAL CALORIES*

1. P. J. Korytko et al., "Induction of hepatic cytochromes P450 in dogs exposed to a chronic low dose of polychlorinated biphenyls," *Toxicological Sciences* (1999), 47(1): 52–61.
2. W. Rea, "Thermal chamber depuration and physical therapy," in *Chemical Sensitivity,* vol. 4 (Boca Raton, FL: Lewis Publishers, 1996): pp. 2433–79.
3. R. M. Cook and K. A. Wilson, "Removal of pesticide residues from dairy cattle," *Journal of Dairy Science* (1971), 54(5): 712–18.
4. R. M. Cook, "Metabolism of xenobiotics in ruminants. Dieldrin recycling from the blood to the gastro-intestinal tract," *Journal of Agricultural and Food Chemistry* (1970), 18(3): 434–6.
5. G. F. Fries et al., "Effect of activated carbon on elimination of organochlorine pesticides from rats and cows," *Journal of Dairy Science* (1970), 53(11): 1632–7.
6. Ibid.
7. W. Rea, "Nutrient replacement: Alkalization," in *Chemical Sensitivity,* vol. 4 (Boca Raton, FL: Lewis Publishers, 1996), pp. 2563–7.
8. Goldman, "Children—Unique and vulnerable."
9. Chadwick et al., "The effects of age and obesity."
10. L. E. Holt and P. H. Holz, "The black bottle," *Journal of Pediatrics* (1963), 63(2): 306–14.
11. Ibid.
12. S. J. Stohs, "The role of free radicals in toxicity and disease," *Journal of Basic and Clinical Physiology and Pharmacology* (1995), 6(3–4): 205–28.
13. M. S. Desole et al., "Neuronal antioxidant system and MPTP induced oxidative stress in the striatum and brain stem of the rat," *Pharmacology, Biochemistry, and Behavior* (1995), 51(4): 581–92.
14. Cheraskin, "Antioxidants in health and disease."
15. Moor de Burgos et al., "Blood vitamin and lipid levels."
16. Rea, "Nutritional status and pollutant overload."
17. Ibid.
18. Guengerich, "Influence of nutrients."
19. S. D. Phinney et al., "Reduced adipose 18:3 omega 3 with weight loss by very low calorie dieting," *Lipids* (1990), 25(12): 798–806.
20. The American Dietetic Association, "Fibre Facts: Soluble Fiber & Heart Disease," (2002) www.eatright.com/nfs/nfs88.html.
21. M. von Ardenne, "Oxygen multistep therapy: Physiological and technical foundations" (Stuttgart/New York: George Thieme Verlag, 1990).
22. Rea, "Thermal chamber depuration."

CHAPTER 15: THE BODY RESTORATION PLAN DIET

1. Cheraskin, "Antioxidants in health and disease."
2. W. Rea, "Nutritional Replacement," in *Chemical Sensitivity,* vol. 4 (Boca Raton, FL: Lewis Publishers, 1996), pp. 2541–684.
3. Department of Health, "Dietary Reference Values."
4. Center for Food Safety and Applied Nutrition, Office of Plant and Dairy Foods and Beverages, *Total Diet Study* (Rockville, MD: U.S. Food and Drug Administration, 2002), Market Baskets 98-2, 98-3, 98-4, 99-1.

CHAPTER 16: TYPICAL QUESTIONS AND USEFUL ANSWERS

1. Moor de Burgos et al., "Blood vitamin and lipid levels."
2. R. V. Patwardhan et al., "Effects of caffeine on plasma free fatty acids, urinary cate-cholamines, and drug binding," *Clinical Pharmacology and Therapeutics* (1980), 28(3): 398–403.
3. Hovinga et al., "Environmental exposure and lifestyle predictors."
4. Alleva et al., "Statement from the work session on environmental endocrine-disrupting chemicals."
5. L. S. Birnbaum, "Endocrine effects of prenatal exposure to PCBs, dioxins, and other xenobiotics: implications for policy and future," *Environmental Health Perspectives* (1994), 102(Aug.): 676–9.
6. L. Brabin and B. J. Brabin, "The cost of successful adolescent growth and development in girls in relation to iron and vitamin A status," *American Journal of Clinical Nutrition* (1992), 55(5): 955–8.
7. T. Baptista et al., "Antipsychotic drugs and reproductive hormones: Relationship to body weight regulation," *Pharmacology, Biochemistry, and Behavior* (1999), 62(3): 409–17.

CHAPTER 17: MAXIMIZE YOUR FITNESS

1. Hu et al., "Comparisons of serum testosterone and corticosterone"; M. Lafontan and M. Berlan, "Fat cell adrenergic receptors and the control of white and brown cell function," *Journal of Lipid Research* (1993), 34(7): 1057–91.
2. Miller and Mumford, "Obesity."
3. N. L. Keim et al., "Effect of exercise and dietary restraint on energy intake of reduced obese women," *Appetite* (1996), 26: 55–70.

4. J. L. Thompson et al., "Effects of diet and diet-plus-exercise programs on resting metabolic rate: a meta-analysis," *International Journal of Sport Nutrition* (1996), 6: 41–61.

5. Ibid.

6. D. L. Ballor et al., "Resistance weight training during caloric restriction enhances lean body weight maintenance," *American Journal of Clinical Nutrition* (1988), 47: 19–25.

Index

285

insecticides, 98, 134, 256, 264. *See also*
pesticides
insect repellents, 131, 137, 246
insulin, 65, 151, 264
intelligence, 19
iodine, 104
iron, 104, 183

ketosis, 13
kidney damage, 171

lamb, 197
lasagne, 96
lead, 117, 258. *See also* heavy metals
leeks, *211*
lemons, 186, *213*
lentils, *206*
lettuce, 94, *204–5*
L-5 hydroxytryptophan, 154, *184*
lice treatments, 130, 137
lime, *204, 213*
lindane, 39–40, 83
linseed oil. *See* flaxseed oil
lipid supplements, 170–71
liver, 167
low-fat foods, 92, 109

magnesium, 59, 104, 157, *183*, 229
margarine, 148, 199, *216*
marmalade, 95, 112, *214*
mattresses, 131
meat, 154, 196–97, 201–2, 223
chemical contamination of, 35, 97, 111,
112, *203, 208–9*
cooking, 112, 187
organic, 97, 102, 103–4, 105, 109, 148–49
religious restrictions, 225–26
medicines, 21, 31, 35, 38, 130
megestrol, 38
melons, *213*
menopause, 229–30
menstrual cycle, 50
menu planning, 188–99
mercury, 258
metabolism, 47, 48, 52, *54–57*, 69–70, 121, 264
methionine, 154, 170, *184*

methyl mercury, 258
microwave cookery, 112, 345
milk, 19, 92, 109, 186, 197, *215*, 245
milk thistle, 172, *185*
minerals, 48, 55, 67, 155, 163, 264
deficiencies, 59–60, 155–57, 250
in foods, 73, 104
supplements, 120, 156–57, 165, 167–68,
172, 182, *183*
mint, 138, *217*
moisturizers, 129
mood changes, 229, 232
moving into a new house, 224–25
MTBE, 116
multivitamins. *See* vitamin supplements
muscles, 229
damaged by chemicals, 66, 69, 161
mushrooms, *204, 211*
mustard, 186, *205*

National Health and Nutritional Examination
Survey III, 59
nausea, 159
nectarines, 196, *213*
nerve gas, 257
New Diet Revolution (Atkins), 13
nits, 130
noodles, *203, 206*
norepinephrine, 264
nutrients, 48, 55, 264
nuts, 96–97, 146, 147, 148–49, 154, 198, *216*,
223

oats, 103, 165, 178, *203, 205*
obesity, 9, 162, 230. *See also* body, fat
percentage
caused by chemicals, 63–64, 81, 150–51,
158–59
cost to health services, 10–11
as an epidemic, 7, 11–12, *12*, 14, 27–28, 72
office workers, 133
okra, *211*
olive oil, 198, *216*
omega-3 and omega-6 oil, 147–49, 170, *184*,
229
supplements, 227